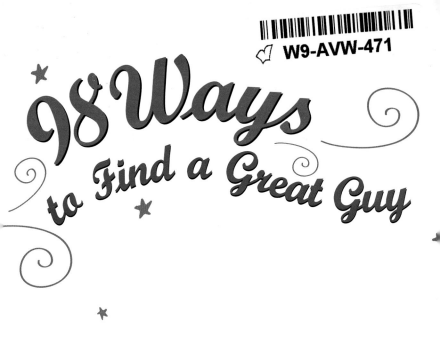

98 Ways to Find a Great Guy

Elizabeth Hazel Paulson

Skyhorse Publishing

Skyhorse Publishing books may be purchased in bulk at
special discounts for sales promotion, corporate gifts,
fund-raising, or educational purposes. Special editions can
also be created to specifications. For details, contact the
Special Sales Department, Skyhorse Publishing, 555 Eighth
Avenue, Suite 903, New York, NY 10018 or
info@skyhorsepublishing.com.

www.skyhorsepublishing.com

10 9 8 7 6 5 4 3 2 1

Library of Congress Cataloging-in-Publication Data

Paulson, Elizabeth.
  98 ways to find a great guy / Elizabeth Paulson.
     p. cm.
  ISBN 978-1-60239-942-6 (pbk. : alk. paper)
  1. Dating (Social customs)--Humor. 2. Man-woman
relationships--Humor. I. Title. II. Title: Ninety-eight ways to
find a great guy.
  PN6231.D3P38 2010
  818'.602--dc22

                          2009039491

Printed in China

TO MY MOM AND SISTER.
AND TO ALL MY EX-BOYFRIENDS.
I COULDN'T HAVE DONE IT WITHOUT YOU,
YOU LITTLE SCAMPS.

FOREWORD

CONGRATULATIONS! *This book has landed itself in your hot little hands!* Put on some lip gloss and pucker up, because you are about to kiss your single days goodbye.

Perhaps you bought this book for yourself. (Smart girl!) Or perhaps some concerned friend bought it for you because she's sick of you whining about being single. (Don't be too hard on her. She did the right thing. Someday you'll be laughing about this—most likely on a double date when the guys have gone up to the bar for drinks.) Or maybe your mom got this for you because she's not getting any younger and she'd like some grandchildren before she's dead. (That's classic Mom!)

How ever you came by this little tome, fear not, gentle reader: Singledom's reign of terror will soon be at an end.

You have before you a collection of boyfriend-finding adventures. Because what is the path to love if not an adventure? I've travelled to the docks in Brooklyn, cliffs of the Irish coast, and wilderness of Alaska. I've worked factory jobs, retail jobs, searched darkest basements, and spent hours watching guys play video games, all in pursuit of the elusive boy-friend. Throughout every caper, I learned from my experiences, nursed wounds (and quite a bit of scotch), and took notes. Every strategy in this book works, though they may not all work for you. But don't worry. For every "In ending this relationship, I'm doing what's best for you" there's an "I'll do the dishes after I massage your feet" waiting around the next corner. Try a bit of everything and even if you don't always pull in a boyfriend for your trouble, you'll have some great stories. You'll find that you can be brave and clever and fabulous, that you can navigate the world of men with wit and grace. And believe me, that will make you even more attractive. They won't stand a chance.

Each of my book's five sections takes into consideration your budget, chances, level of desperation, recklessness, or inclination toward going out and putting forth some effort. So see how you feel on a particular day and plot accordingly. Enjoy your time alone with this book because soon you'll be a very, very busy lady. Happy hunting!

—Elizabeth Paulson
New York City

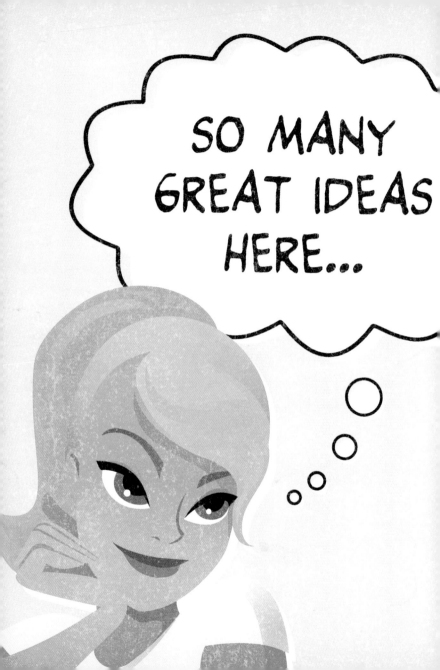

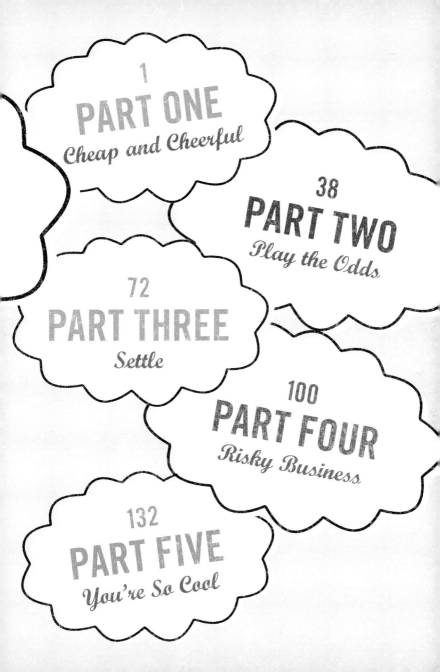

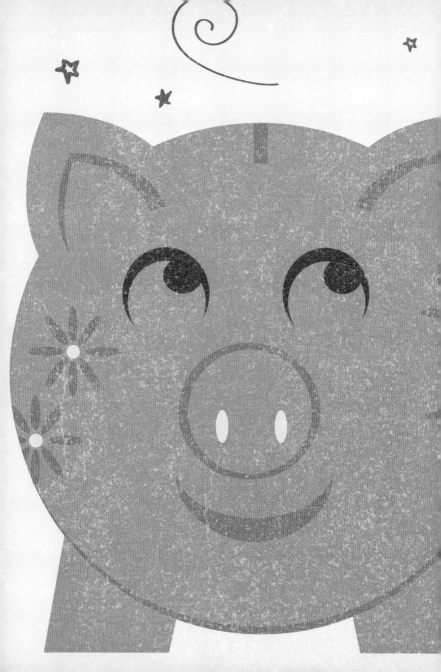

Cheap and Cheerful

YOU'RE ALREADY INVESTING YOUR TIME
AND GOOD FAITH IN THIS BOYFRIEND-
FINDING LARK. NO ONE EVER SAID IT HAS
TO COST YOU MONEY, TOO.

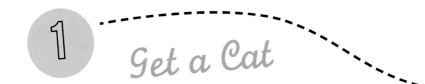

1 Get a Cat

PUT CAT IN TREE.
CALL FIRE DEPARTMENT.
APPLY LIPSTICK.
SHAKE MARTINIS.

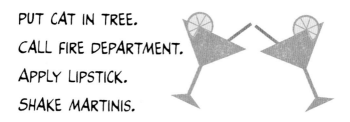

Or, for the more responsible types:
Say you have a cat. Claim that cat is up a tree. Call fire department. Apply lipstick. Be bereft when little Bill Masterton Trophy Winner Ken Daneyko[*] is nowhere to be found. Take solace in the cutest firefighter the station sends.

Pros: He's big, he's strong, and he'd run into a burning building for you!

Cons: He'd run into a burning building for anyone, even your fictitious cat.

[*]Of course you named him after your favorite hockey player!

2. Get a Pen Pal

"How did we meet? **Well, it's a** super-cute story. I was studying in Trondheim and there was this really adorable tour guide at Nidaros Cathedral. I kept going again and again, and at the end, I slipped him my email address. We'd been writing to each other ever since then, and last year we decided to take the plunge. Now Knut's moved in with me!"

Little does Knut know that the entire time your epistolary relationship was blossoming into love, you made the rounds with every guy within a ten-block radius of your house. And you completely abandoned the gym. And took up smoking. And drugs. And you sent about 12,000 drunken text messages to other guys, threw up in front of a third of them, went to jail twice, and did countless other hideously embarrassing and unattractive things. But in your correspondence you never reported anything but clean living and fidelity. On paper, you're the perfect mate and he's lucky to have you. Enjoy!

Pros: You can have your lutefisk and eat it, too.

Cons: He probably did the exact same thing to you. Good luck with your open and honest relationship!

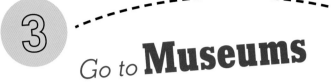

Go to **Museums**

Museums are great because if you find a guy there, he's likely to be employed, decently dressed, and quite possibly a cultured gentleman. **(Or looking to pick up chicks.)** Be sure to wear high heels, so your prospects can hear you click-clacking down the marble halls. It's also handy to find a bench so you can cross and uncross your legs as you contemplate *The Night Watch* or anything else grand in scope. And never, ever get the audio commentary—you don't want anything separating you from your future boyfriend—even if the insights on Monet's parent and adolescent haystacks are fascinating. Then, start perusing the collection.

Medieval armor, Pompeii, and the Egyptian wing attract the men. If you find yourself in a museum without the equivalent of these, do what you can with actual paintings. Stick to modern art—anything past the Impressionists and you're fine (though they do like van Gogh). Abstract Expressionism always delights, as does Pop Art. Dada is right up their alley, not surprisingly. Surrealism? They'll go for

4

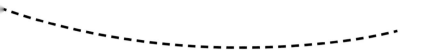

seconds. And anything postmodern and vulgar will always attract our gentlemen friends. *The Physical Impossibility of Death in the Mind of Someone Living*? Find it and then say some witty quote from *Jaws* to the banker-on-his-lunch-break-type standing next to you. Ta-da! You've got yourself a date for Friday.

Pros: It's good for you!

Cons: Some of that stuff will give you nightmares.

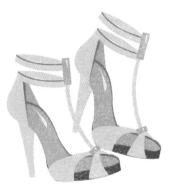

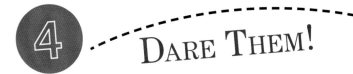

4 DARE THEM!

Men love a good dare. Use this to your advantage. **When a guy asks for your** number, write it down and throw it in the trash. This, of course, presents a challenge to the man, and, since he's a man, he won't be able to resist digging out that piece of paper, calling you, and asking you out. Would he have called you if you hadn't done that little trick? I don't think so! When has anyone ever called you after you've said, "Sure, here's my number! Let me type it into your phone for you! I've also included my work phone, fax, parents' number in Pennsylvania, and dog walker, just in case"? Never.

So this is the approach a smart girl takes when she's out and someone slides up to her, makes about a minute and a half's worth of conversation, and then asks for her number:

"Why?" you ask the unlucky gent.

"Because I wanna take you out for a beverage sometime," he replies.

"Uh-huh, right. I'm sure if I give you my number, you'll think about me all of tomorrow and then call me the day after," you say.

"I will! Honestly!" he protests.

"Riiiiiight," you say.

"Would I ask for your number if I didn't want to see you again?" he asks.

"It's usually the surest way to ensure it," you reply tartly. This goes on for quite a while, giving you ample time to assess the poor man who ran afoul of you.

If he seems like a jerk, he gets the number of your least favorite ex-boyfriend, assuming you remember it, or else he gets a number that you've just made up. If he seems like a nice guy who actually might be a keeper, apologize, put your hand on his arm, and say something like, "Oh it's so tough in the city. I'm afraid I can't help being a little jaded. Most guys are such jerks, you know." And voilà, you've explained your hideous behavior and complimented him all in one fell swoop. As he finishes entering your number in his phone, throw in one more, "For all the good it will do you. It's not like you'll use it!" with a twinkling little laugh. Then turn on your fabulous little heels and leave him staring after your swishy hair, besotted and with more resolve to actually use your number.

Pros: He's going to call you! He really will!

Cons: The story of your first meeting will forever feature you in the role of harpy.

5

USE YOUR SMUG MARRIED FRIENDS AS HEADHUNTERS

Let's be honest: you haven't heard from your best friend since she got married.

And it's not the first time this has happened. All your friends seem to lose interest in you as soon as they're married. But they gain interest in one important thing: the institution. Now that they've seen the light, they want you to, too. So humor them. When they tell you how great their life is now and that you should really settle down, tell them to be on the search for you. They'll think themselves very mature and benevolent, finding poor dear little single you a mate almost (but not quite) as nice as theirs is.

Pros: Soon you'll be married!

Cons: Married couples don't feel like they need to shut the door when they go to the bathroom. Gross.

6
DRESS LIKE A SLUT ON HALLOWEEN

It's secretly how you want to dress anyway, so live it up on the one socially acceptable day to do it. You'll turn heads, hearts, and, if you go as Zombie Roller Girl, maybe even stomachs. Just try to be a tad more creative than your competition. Sticking a pair of bunny ears, devil horns, or a nurse hat on top of you dressed like a slut won't distinguish you from the masses. Go the extra mile and you'll be going the extra mile with whichever eligible ghoul you choose.

Pros: All your potential future boyfriends will be in good moods, since they'll be dressed as women, which is how they want to dress anyway.

Cons: It's discouraging to know, right off the bat, that he's got nicer legs than you.

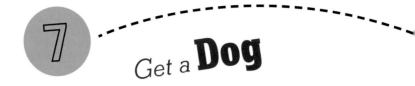

Get a **Dog**

Just as you're allowed to approach any random person walking down the street who happens to have a dog, your dog is allowed to approach any random person! Get a dog and you'll open yourself up to a whole new social life. You'll be more approachable. Guys won't be able to resist your adorable little (or big) puppy at the end of the leash. You'll meet attractive local dog owners at puppy classes and the dog run. You and the dog will be quite the man-catching team! And if all else fails, you can teach him to play dead in front of attractive single guys. He'll trot up and fall over right in front of the target. Then you can quickly run to see what the matter is. Thinking your darling pooch dead, you can wail and look, with big teary eyes, to your unsuspecting man for help. After he awkwardly comforts you for as long as necessary, up will spring your dog and you'll all have a miracle to talk about over drinks later.

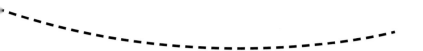

Pros: You'll have someone who is always glad to see you, who'll protect you from nightmares (I told you not to look too closely at the scary paintings), and a warm body next to you at night.

Cons: If you have that, you don't really need a boyfriend now, do you?

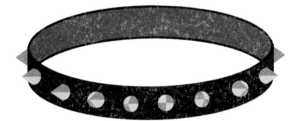

8

Join the Kickball League and Wear a Rugby Shirt

"Really? You're going to join the kickball league? That's cool, I guess, seeing as how you're a girl and all and league rules require at least two girls on the field at all times. So yeah, great, but don't expect us to give you any special treatment just because you're a girl. Okay? Good. Let's never talk about how you're a girl again. What's that? You know the manager of that bar and you can get them to sponsor us? That's awesome. And hey, at practice today you showed some mad skills. You wear gym shorts and a rugby shirt, just like us guys do. I don't feel alienated by you at all. And your hair in that ponytail is kind of hot. Or is it a pigtail? You don't know the difference? Ha ha, me neither. I guess we'll have to ask one of our female coworkers who are all too stuck up and afraid to break a nail to play kickball. They're not like you at all. You're cool. Oh, you drink beer, too? Man, that's crazy—you're just

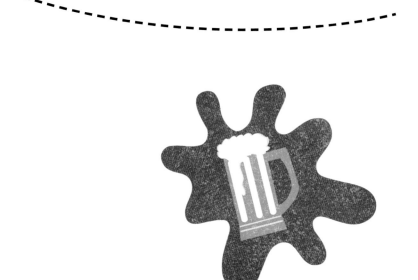

like one of the guys! Wanna hang out this weekend and discuss strategy for next Tuesday's match against the team sponsored by Hooters?"

Pros: You'll get as many guys as the league can lob at you.

Cons: You're a grown woman playing a game meant for children on elementary school playgrounds.

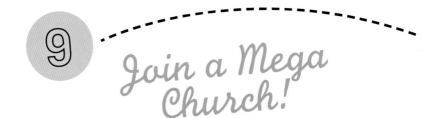

9

Join a Mega Church!

Behind Jim there was Tammy Faye, Joel has Victoria, and Rick Warren has, um, Mrs. Warren. Three power couples associated with mega churches: big, non-denominational Christian stadiums devoted to loving Jesus and finding happiness in this world. There's at least one in your area; put on something nice, make your hair bigger, and go find it. You will soon have a place in the singles twenty-to-twenty-five Bible study group, or the singles twenty-six-to-thirty Bible study group, or the singles thirty-one-to-thirty-six Bible study group. Lots of new friends to make! And you'll have so many chances to give back to the less fortunate on many organized volunteer trips. Getting a boyfriend and building someone a house? Not bad for a day's work.

Are you flexible on religion and think feminism is overrated? If so, go conservative. Be born again and your fellow parishioners will promptly set about finding just the right guy for you. And what a right guy he will be! These men have their priorities in order—he'll have a sensible job, cushy bank account, a nice car, and his own house. All you have to do is move in! And, since sex before marriage is deeply frowned upon by these types, you'll be walking down that mile-long aisle in no time.

Pros: He won't cheat on you, but if he does, you both know he's going to hell. Ha!

Cons: Lots of cooking and cleaning and child-rearing and keeping opinions to yourself.

10

Be the **Liaison to the IT Department**

Help improve your *division's relationship with the IT department one help-desk call at a time.* It's not improbable that you're known best among the computer geeks as the girl who got into work one morning, called IT, and said her computer was broken. They might remember your proud indignation when they asked you if you'd turned on your computer yet. "Obviously," you said. When they "fixed" your computer by turning on the monitor, they probably recall how you scowled, waited a beat, and then said, "Did you know you can pour a whole cup of coffee on your keyboard and nothing bad will happen?" And then they got to see you later that day when your keyboard stopped working. What a treat you were!

Not to worry. Modern IT guys, believe it or not, have a sense of humor. You might have a reputation for being a perfect jerk to them, but if you have the good grace to know when you're beaten, you'll be fine. Volunteer to be your department's IT problem coordinator. Or whatever term they might use for that. You'll have every reason to flirt with those boys in the computer room. Trust me, they'll think you're amazing.

It'd probably be worth your time to learn the terms "router" and "modem" and "mouse." Anyway, say you'll make the phone calls to your nice new friends downstairs and start uploading yourself into their hearts.

Pros: Someone who'll deal with anything you own that has a plug.

Cons: They're not much for conversation beyond telling you where to plug it.

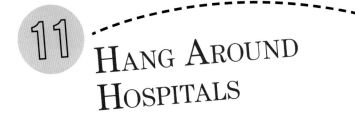

11 HANG AROUND HOSPITALS

MEET DOCTORS!

GET IN TOUCH WITH YOUR OWN MORTALITY!

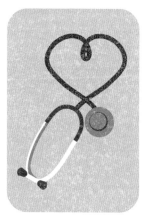

Doctors are very busy and important,
so if you want to meet one, you'll have to go to them.
But first, watch a lot of soap operas so you'll know
how to behave in a hospital. You will see how it's
important to always be very dressed up, occasionally

sneak in and unplug someone from life support, and fake a death certificate.

Then, in order to not seem like a Münchausen syndrome patient, you should probably get a job in the hospital before you start camping out there.* Be a candy striper, sell Mylar balloons in the gift shop, be the chaplain, or go through seven years of medical school! From then on, it's just a waiting game to see who will be the first doctor to diagnose you as date-positive.

Pros: A doctor! The crown jewel in the boyfriend crown!

Cons: MRSA infection.

*Unless you actually are a Münchausen syndrome patient, in which case, sit back, take another hit of arsenic, and get ready to meet Dr. Right.

12

Have a Chance Subway Encounter

Why does the Internet exist if not to give us a second chance **after a missed connection?** There are so many websites out there where you can try to reconnect with the guy whose name you didn't manage to get, either on the subway that morning or at a bar the other night, that it's foolish not to use them. Either put up a posting about yourself, make something up, or browse postings from guys and see if you don't fit any of the descriptions.

Pros: It's cheaper than online dating!

Cons: You might have to dye your hair red. But you needed a change anyway, and if he's got a redhead on his mind, then you be that redhead.

13

Play Frisbee... Or Look Like You Do

Dude, you toss? That's awesome! Find a park, follow the smell of unwashed men and the sound of pukashell necklaces bouncing against grimy collarbones, and have your pick of the Frisbee boys.

Pros: You'll never be frustrated at him for sitting around on the couch all day.

Cons: His attention span is as short as your tolerance for his moochy friends.

14

WORK ON A POLITICAL CAMPAIGN!

Where else can you meet dozens of young, idealistic, and passionate people, just like you? And after three months on the campaign trail, there will be barely showered, exhausted, and overweight-from-too-much-fast-food people, just like you! Finally, a guy who shares your same strong interest in issues, doing good, and selfless service toward one's country! And one who won't tell you that he thinks you're disgusting, because he's gotten just as gross as you have.

Try to stick to your own age and rank. The governor may come out the worst when he trifles with the cute young staffer, what with his career being destroyed and all, but darn if that doesn't end the girl's political ambitions, too. So keep to your fellow college-goers, or your direct supervisor if you absolutely must have some scandal.

Wait until the next twenty-hour day. You've been up since five making pies for the candidate's wife to give out at the next school event, and your

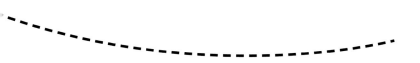

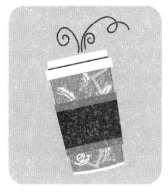

target has been chauffeuring the candidate around the great state of Iowa for the past seventeen hours. Invite him to come blow off some steam at the local watering hole, and soon you'll be giving the people of Des Moines something far more interesting than the campaign to talk about.

Pros: You'll have worked together to achieve an amazing, world-changing goal! (You getting a boyfriend, obviously.)

Cons: All that campaign food can really kill a guy's sex drive.

Go to AA and NA Meetings

One day at a time, darling, and you're sure to find a sensitive guy who's willing to admit he's got a problem. And how great is that? A guy willing to admit he's got a problem! For that reason alone, attending Alcoholics Anonymous and Narcotics Anonymous meetings will be a breath of fresh air!

To keep your sanity as you begin a life of half-hearted clean living, you'll need to go to both meetings so you'll get two boyfriends—one in front of whom you shouldn't drink and the other in front of whom you shouldn't do hard drugs. At least you can keep half your vices at all times. And don't forget, the more meetings you go to, the more free coffee and snacks you'll get! Think of the savings on meals and caffeine.

Pros: It's anonymous!

Cons: You're so much less fun at parties now that you've pretended to quit drinking and doing drugs.

16. BE PRETTY AND SOFT AND SMELL LIKE FRUIT

It's that easy! **Men love it** when women are pretty and soft and smell like fruit. All you have to do is follow a simple new beauty regimen consisting of keeping yourself constantly exfoliated and slathered with lotion. Also, avoid anything that might cause skin to roughen, like walking or doing things with your hands. Keep a supply of magazines on hand to tell you what's pretty from month to month. If you can hit the sacred trifecta, you'll have someone to keep you in L'Occitane products for the rest of your life.

Pros: You'll be pretty and soft and smell like fruit!

Cons: Hard to maintain.

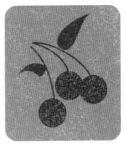

17 Shamelessly Write Down Your Email Address

As mother always said, "Never bother with a sniper rifle when a shotgun will do." This is the theory behind shamelessly writing down your email address on every credit card receipt at every restaurant or bar where an attractive man has waited upon you. It's a broadcast approach to man-hunting and one with which many women aren't always comfortable. But, like applying liquid eyeliner, or going to the gynecologist, it gets easier every time. Soon enough, it's second nature.

Start by sheepishly admitting to your friends that you're going to try this new method. They'll either tell you to get a life or help you identify candidates worthy of your contact info. Either way, they'll know what you're up to and won't be so embarrassed for you at the end of the meal. Then, get scribbling.

It's best to mix it up a bit. Going to the same place repeatedly can make for confusion. When he calls and identifies himself as "the guy from that bar, The Redhead, the one where you ate all that flatbread" your job is to play it cool, but not as cool as saying, "Great, were you Tuesday drinks, Thursday dinner, or Sunday pre-dinner drinks?"

Needless to say, you've got to avoid doing this at your favorite haunts. Pick the places you couldn't live without and exempt yourself from your receipt routine there. You don't want to come in the next night and be waited on by the guy who had no interest in your interest. Talk about leaving a bad taste in your mouth! Know what restaurants are sacred to you because nothing should jeopardize your ability to go there and eat your heart out as often as you please, no matter how sure you are that your regular waiter is single and quite possibly into you.

Pros: If it doesn't work, you'll have the opportunity to try lots of new places! Lots . . .

Cons: You've bagged yourself a waiter, oh dear. Chances are he's an actor. See #80.

18

Join the March Madness Pool

OBVIOUSLY, YOU'RE NOT GOING TO FILL OUT YOUR BRACKET YOURSELF.

That's what your father, brother-in-law, or friend's boyfriend is for. Unless you actually know something about basketball, in which case, go for it! No matter how much better you are than your competition, though, your job is to act as girlie as possible about it and, whenever someone congratulates you on your steady ascension, giggle and say something like, "Well, my method of choosing winners based on how many consonants are in the mascot's name never fails!" This will severely annoy some of your competitors, but they're probably girls or men who take the whole thing too seriously. You don't want to date either of those. The important thing is, you're in the game and you're getting noticed. Now go out and win it, sport.

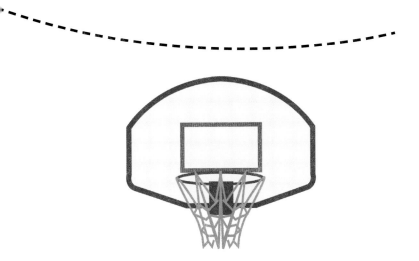

Pros: Some of these pools involve real money! A simple five dollar investment could mean winnings of tens of dollars AND the love of your life.

Cons: You'll have to feign interest in college basketball long enough for your eyes not to glaze over when Hunky McFreethrow starts talking about it. Don't ever let on that you'd rather be talking about the latest issue of the *Utne Reader*. And you might have to forfeit your winnings to whomever filled out your answer sheet.

ACCUSE HIM OF BEING GAY

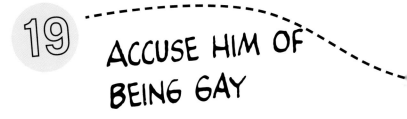

If he says he's just not that into you, **don't lose heart.** Keep this ace up your sleeve: "It's because you're gay, isn't it? I knew it! You're so gay! Well, I feel a lot better now, knowing you're *totally* a homosexual and don't like women! *Phew!*"

Find a big enough homophobe and he'll do anything to prove you wrong. Even date you.

Pros: You've entered into a fear-based relationship and you've got the upper hand! Finally!

Cons: He might actually be gay.

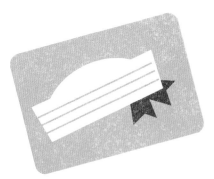

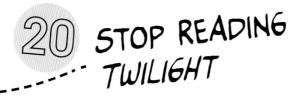

20 STOP READING TWILIGHT

Or *Harry Potter*, or *The Thorn Birds*, or *The Prophet*, or whatever it is the kids today are reading. Sure there's nothing you'd like to do better than go straight home and find out what happens next, but guess what? Neither Edward Cullen nor Cardinal de Bricassart is going to keep you warm at night. Especially not Edward. And the sad truth is that you can't be seen reading anything of this sort in public. Men simply won't take you seriously. Even if they're standing around with a copy of *Maxim* or John Grisham, you're not beyond reproach. It's one of those cruel injustices of the universe.

Pros: You'll have more time to read the intelligent literary fiction that's been piling up on your bedside table. Or, even better, you'll have more time to read what your future boyfriend would read! Grab a *Sports Illustrated* or the *Wall Street Journal*, or flip through a Calvin and Hobbes coffee-table book.

Cons: You won't be able to make people think you're better than them by comparing the movie to the book in your usual disdainful manner.

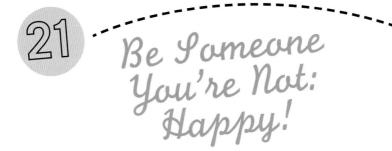

21

Be Someone You're Not: Happy!

No one likes a bitter girl. **Even if you're** eating yourself up inside because you've just lost your best friend to marriage, or you've gained five pounds overnight, or work is unbearable, or you're still single, don't let that get the best of you. Or let it get the best of you, but keep that hidden way down deep inside. Instead, be the most superficially happy person you can possibly be. Men, even dower Schopenhauer-types, are attracted to happiness. And, as much as you'd hate to admit it, pretending to be happy is half the battle! Pretty soon you'll be smiling and behaving like a decent human being automatically, with no thought of how tiring it is for you. If you need a jumpstart, watch the movie *Enchanted*. It's foolproof.

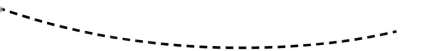

Pros: This is a transferable skill. Everyone wants to give the job, extra serving of cake, lower interest rate, or upgraded hotel room to the happy girl. Not to that snarky crone next to her.

Cons: Someday you're going to snap, and let's hope it's not in public. Or in front of your husband and kids. Let's hope you die long before your repressed angst surfaces.

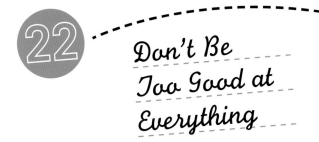

22 Don't Be Too Good at Everything

We've all been there—you're out at the grain *elevator, standing with your sisters in the back of the truck, shoveling the grain into the auger.* You're doing a great job! The mice running across your feet don't bother you a bit, and you're keeping the pace steady so that you don't clog the aforementioned auger. All of a sudden, up comes Michael Stone, the cool city-boy nephew of the farmer down the road. He offers to help. He's super cute, so you ignore the fact that he's from Minneapolis and has no idea what he's doing. He starts doing everything wrong. The next thing you know, there's spilled grain everywhere and the darned auger is jammed and you're shoving Michael away because he's only screwing things up. He leaves, defeated and embarrassed, and your chances with him are shot.

Point is, a lot of men go for women who are nearly self-sufficient and who could almost get by without them. It's great when you know how to do things, but just a little worse or a teeny bit more slowly than he would do it. You'll be a great team! With him carrying a touch over 51 percent of the load. Assuming it's a physical load—like if you're hauling feed sacks into the barn. Any sort of psychological burden and you're on your own, sweetie.

Pros: It's fun to make them think they're superior to you. Such a warm, smug feeling in your heart.

Cons: You could get any given task completed twice as fast if you weren't waiting around for him to show you how to do it poorly and incorrectly.

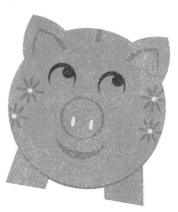

23 Have a Good Wing Woman

Almost as hard to find as a good boyfriend is a good wing woman—a girl who will go out with you and keep your goals in mind. She is someone who is endlessly entertaining on her own but who won't bat an eyelash before seizing the chance to engage in conversation with a potential boyfriend for you. Once you find her, don't let her go, for she shall be the most valuable thing you have in your boyfriend-finding arsenal.

A good wing woman is hard to find primarily because a good wing woman is not single. And once you're scouting non-single territory, you'll be hard pressed to find anyone willing to go back to the dark, desperate world of single life with you. Why would she want to? She'd have a much better time doing something with her husband or boyfriend and not getting depressed by stale old you. What if your singledom is contagious and she goes home to find herself dumped? So not worth it!

But, she does exist, really. Like Kipling's "Thousandth Man," the giant squid, or a cabbie willing to take you to JFK at 3:30 on a Friday afternoon, she is out there. You just have to be patient and the right one will come along.

Pros: You have a wing woman, a very best friend, someone to sympathize with you, to take you out when you need a pick-me-up, someone who understands everything about you.

Cons: She, even better than a dog, fulfills so many of the requirements you're looking for in a boyfriend, you could do worse than give up the quest once you've found her.

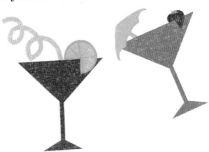

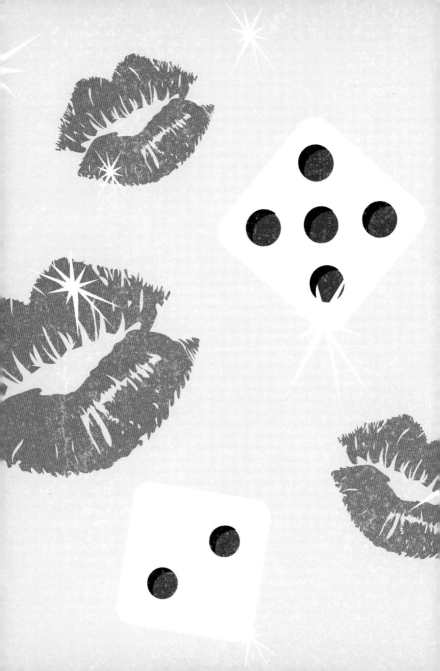

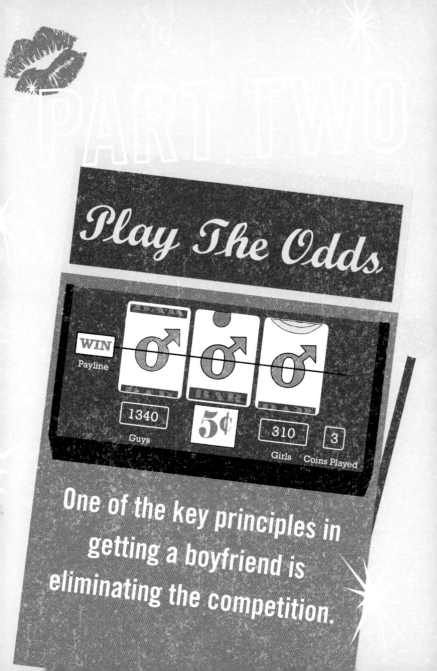

PART TWO

Play The Odds

WIN
Payline

1340
Guys

5¢

310
Girls

3
Coins Played

One of the key principles in getting a boyfriend is eliminating the competition.

KA-BOOM!!!...

24 GO TO COMIC-CON

WHAT THE EFF IS COMIC-CON, YOU SAY?
WELL LISTEN UP, LOSER. IF YOU'RE LOOKING
FOR AN IT MAN WITH AN UNTOUCHED BANK
ACCOUNT AND A GREAT BIG BASEMENT
IN HIS PARENTS' HOUSE, AND YOU DON'T
MIND IF HE SOMETIMES WEARS A CAPE,
COMIC-CON IS YOUR GEEK-CHIC PARADISE.

The convention is held twice a year—in San Diego and New York—so there's really no excuse not to go. And the prep for this one could not be easier: simply bring your two X chromosomes and you're all set. If you're looking to increase your chances even further, go one more step and dress like a comic book character. Are you blonde? Get yourself a headband and go as Gwen Stacy! Redheaded? Why, you could be MJ! Take your pick, brunettes: do you want to be Lois Lane or Wonder Woman? If you're looking for instantaneous proposals, traipse around in a gold metal bikini. At the very least, you'll make these boys' lives. And a lot of blogs.

Pros: You're the coolest thing that's ever happened to this guy since he learned the Konami Code. When's the last time a guy worshipped you? You can be his Kryptonite! Such power! Drink it in!

Cons: And you thought these things smelled bad on the outside. . . . Hygiene could be an issue.

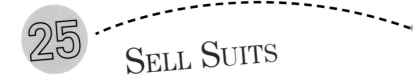

25

SELL SUITS

There's no better way to find a man in a suit than to sell it to him. And you'll get commission too.

No matter how appealing the Victoria's Secret employee discount is, you must forget the instant gratification of free underwear when you're looking for an employer, and remember what you're really shopping for. Work at a men's store—make sure the clothes are slim-fit and modern, no pleated trousers here, thank you very much—and you'll not only save money on clothes you don't need anyway, you can screen for a new Mr. Right to try on for size.

Single men—and you'll quickly learn to identify them—need the most help clothes shopping. They'll come in the store, eyes darting nervously, their big sweaty hands pawing whatever pile of sweaters happens to be in front of them, and, if left unattended, end up leaving with two pairs of socks and a belt. You can't let this happen. It isn't fair to them, your store, or your selfish secret motivations to find a man.

Don't forget: it's your job to make the first move. After all, they do need to know your name in case the sizes aren't right, and they will need to tell you if there's anything else you can get for them. Your clients will pick up on your ability to match colors, iron shirts, and differentiate between business casual and beachwear and cling to you for the rest of your shift. By that time you'll know what kind of guy you've got, and if he's the one for you. And when you walk him over to the cash registers, you smile brightly and say, "I've attached my card in case you need anything." (Insert smoldering look here.)

Works every time, *mes amies*. Every time.

Pros: Every day, a new shipment.

Cons: Every day, a new shipment . . . of shirts to steam and boxers to stock and sale items to mark down.

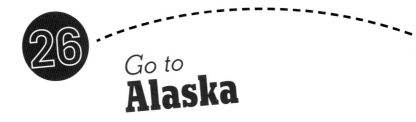

26

Go to
Alaska

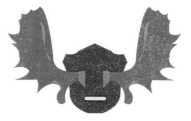

In fact, go to Alaska anyway. It's a great place to get over a break-up. **You can divide your time** between visualizing the ex-boyfriend abandoned on a glacier and visualizing yourself on a date with one of the myriad wilderness hunks on offer in the Last Frontier State. It's only a matter of time before you become obsessed with the idea of fleeing New York (or New Wherever) for the big sky desolation of Alaska—assuming, of course, you could start your new life with a taciturn and capable mountain man beside you. But how does a girl find one?

Luckily, there's the *Talkeetna Bachelor Society's Male Order Catalog.* The good citizens have made it so easy! It provides photographs, ages, and interests of all forty eligible men in the town. Just pick your favorite and write to him. Sure, most look like refugees from a production of *Deliverance: On Ice*, but there are indeed some winners. The lady at the shop who will sell you this catalog will warn you: "The odds are good, but the goods are odd." But come on, when's the last time you went out on the town gold digging and actually found yourself a gold miner? If you're seeking the quiet freezing life, write to our friends in Talkeetna. You know how to field dress a deer and clean a fish, right?

Pros: Long winter nights of hunkering down together in a log cabin, with no one around for miles, fire crackling, coffee on the boil, and solitude.

Cons: Long winter nights of hunkering down together in a log cabin, with no one around for miles, fire crackling, coffee on the boil, and solitude.

Go to a Car Show; Display Some Knowledge of Cars

It's so surprising, so endearing, so hot, in Pretty Woman *when* **Julia Roberts's** character hops into Richard Gere's borrowed Lotus Esprit, slides it into gear, and says it corners like it's on rails. She's a girl! Who can identify car makes and models! And she can drive a manual transmission! And in less than two hours, she's landed a fabulously wealthy, single, and emotionally unavailable dreamboat. Happily ever after!

How can you hope to follow in those tranny-booted footsteps? Instead of running away and becoming a prostitute, brush up on cars! No, it's not as adventurous and the skills aren't as transferable, but it's more impressive at most cocktail parties.

The great thing about cars is that you don't actually have to know a lot about them to seem like you do. Just a few key stats, words, and phrases is all it takes. You're already at a car show, for crying out loud, or at a party where the guys have started talking Italian sports cars versus American muscle cars and your eyes haven't glazed over. That's most of the work done already. And, since guys like to use cars to pick up women, they'll actually care about your opinion and won't sneer when you say cute girl things like:

"I think 'flappy paddle gear box' is just the most adorable term."

"I'll take whichever one has gull-wing or scissor doors!"

"The Jaguar XF is admittedly a fantastic piece of machinery, and certainly a departure from its too-naff predecessors, but I think it's rather derivative of an Aston Martin, at least cosmetically, and if you're buying a Jag because it looks like an Aston, wouldn't you rather just pony up the extra whatever grand for an actual Aston? I don't know. I would. But maybe that's just me!"

Pros: New car smell is even better than new boyfriend smell.

Cons: Careful: if he actually owns a really nice car, he just might be compensating for something.

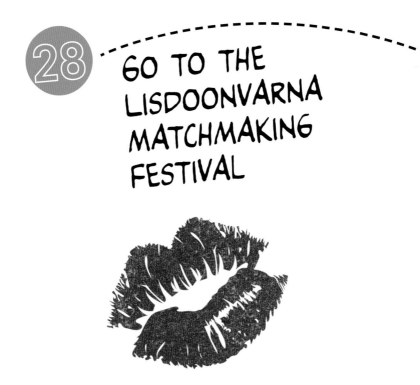

28 GO TO THE LISDOONVARNA MATCHMAKING FESTIVAL

It's not the only matchmaking festival, but it's definitely the most fun.

Lisdoonvarna is a tiny town in Ireland's County Clare, and every year tens of thousands of singles flood the place for five weeks in September and October. Join them! Check in to your hotel, get yourself on Willie Daly's books (he's the resident matchmaker), and sit down for a pint while he sorts someone out for you. Willie's family has been in the matchmaking business for generations, ever since the farmers in the area started having trouble getting wives, so trust him. You can go to the festival dances safe in the knowledge that someone else is handling the problem of your being single. And there's a pretty good chance that you'll be proposed to at least three times before you've even met the guys Willie's selected for you. You won't be able to make a move for the bathroom without dozens of eager men asking for your hand.

Pros: You'll have a boyfriend or husband in plenty of time for going home for Christmas!

Cons: Although the festival attracts bachelors from around the world, there's a good chance you'll get matched with an Irish farmer.

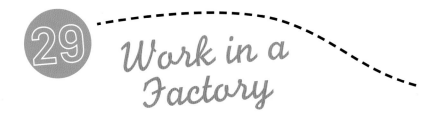

29 Work in a Factory

Okay, so maybe you don't exactly equate Norma Rae with "gets all the best dates," **but hold on a sec and take** a look at your odds: one little (comparatively speaking) you, dozens of burly men. You'd be mad not to drive out to the steel belt and see what's on offer. Working in a factory is great money, will keep you in shape (all that heavy lifting of parts and managing of giant, unruly machines), and it'll give you a shift's worth of access (plus overtime!) to our nation's hardest-working hunks. Sure you're sweaty the whole time, and you're bleeding or bruised from the second you punch in, but compared to Skully, the second shift electro-mechanical engineer, you're a hot little number.

Pros: You get to drive a forklift! Cool.

Cons: Glass-filled nylon has a three-hundred-degree Fahrenheit working temperature. You don't get your fingers back once you mess with that.

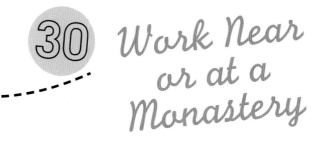

Work Near or at a Monastery

Before you get all scandalized, consider that temptation goes with their territory. It's something all holy men and women struggle with and it's hardly your fault for being the one doing the tempting. You just work there. And if you find that the pickings are even better than at Comic-Con, all the better for everyone! Or you, at least. Who's to say you're not doing them a favor by keeping them from committing to a life that wasn't really right for them? Maybe you're a godsend!

Pros: You'll get to go shopping for all new clothes for him! And once his tonsure grows in, you'll have free reign over his hair! Never have you had this great an opportunity to make your man!

Cons: Aside from making bread, beer, or brandy, he probably doesn't have too many skills.

Work at a
Bait Shop

Fat heads, leeches, small fry, night crawlers, stinkers, suckers—those are just some of the men you'll meet at your cool new job at the bait shop. And you'll learn all about bait, too!

Is there anything that says summer like "part-time job at the bait shop"? No, ma'am. Get a gig slinging chum for fishermen far and wide and you've practically transported yourself into a Bryan Adams song. In no time at all, Jimmy, Matt, Dan, and the rest will be vying for the chance to take you to Shooters for pan-seared walleye cheeks and pull tabs after work.

Feasting and gambling and everything nice await you. All you have to do is hurry up and finish restocking the .380 hollow-points and stacking the prize muskies and other extraordinarily large fish in the front window.

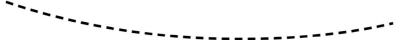

Pros: Get yourself a fisherman and just think of all the time you'll have to yourself!

Cons: There are more dignified ways to go through life than up to your elbows in fish entrails. And that stuff does not come out of denim. Or anything else, for that matter.

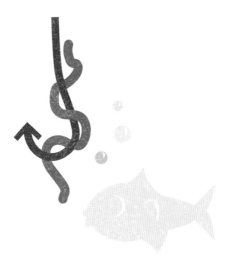

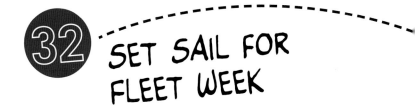

32 SET SAIL FOR FLEET WEEK

More commonly known as "The Week Before Memorial Day Weekend," **Fleet** Week is a very special time for the women of New York City. This is when selected members of the U.S. Armed Forces come to the city to display their might, prowess, strength, and partying ability. There's also something about them doing flyovers and drills on ships to show taxpayers where all their money is going. But that's beside the point.

Whatever the purpose, this glorious influx of men in uniform as far as the eye can see is nothing less than breathtaking. So mark your calendar for next year and plan a trip to New York. Get a nice centrally located hotel and you'll have plenty of reasons to give him for not going back to his ship. For him to drop anchor with you, as it were. To park his dingy in your marina, as the more crass among us would say. To drop his blood stripes on your striped carpet. To hang his cover on your bedpost. Et cetera.

Some of these boys will be pretty rough around the edges. Sailors have that reputation for a reason, you know. They might demand that they get the last potato skin or other bar detritus, reminding you that you sleep under what blanket at night? Yeah, that's right, a blanket of freedom. And who's providing you with that blanket? Yes, he is. So back off and give a marine his due. The trick is to find a group big enough so that you'll meet some creeps, some adorably engaged, and some just rights. At least you're guaranteed great photos of you in their cute little hats.

Fleet Week boys are always impressed when you know which uniforms are which and when you can tell who is senior to whom. Watch a whole bunch of movies like *Saving Private Ryan*, *A Bridge Too Far*, *An Officer and a Gentleman*, *A Few Good Men*, or the entire boxed set of *Band of Brothers* in preparation. Nothing wrong with throwing in *Top Gun* for good measure.

Pros: They'll be so sweet and so polite and call you "ma'am"!

Cons: Who are they calling "ma'am"? Do you really look that old?

33 Be the Psychologist for the NYPD

While being the psychologist for any police department will do, movies and television shows seem to suggest that the NYPD needs your caring ministrations the most. Definitely avoid Boston. You'll just get caught on the periphery of a Scorsese film and honestly, you don't have that kind of time. There's still a healthy male-to-female ratio among New York's finest, so you'll be dealing with lots more troubled men than with women. Revel in the power (and hot dates) to be grabbed. You'll get to wear short skirts and sexy glasses while they reluctantly dribble their hearts out to you. You'll have the personnel files on all of them. You'll be in charge of determining whether they get stuck on desk duty or get to go back to the streets. They need you a lot more than you need them, and many will be happy to do whatever it takes for a glowing report and your seal of "professional" approval.

Pros: Hour after hour of new recruits!

Cons: Medical/workplace/professional ethics. Or whatever.

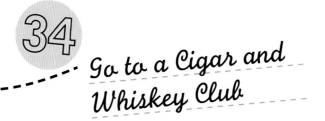

34 · Go to a Cigar and Whiskey Club

Another one of those places where men least expect you! If you have the good taste to like whiskey and can stomach the smell of cigars without throwing up, show off these skills at the local cigar and whiskey place! Grab a girlfriend and your gold card and prepare to bemuse dozens of suits with expense accounts.

More than anywhere else, attitude is important here. Pretend you know what you're doing. Even if you don't know a single malt scotch from a triple distilled whiskey, just order confidently and you will gain the respect of your waiter and your fellow patrons. And if you do know your way around the Glenlivet XXV, good job! There's a pretty good chance you'll be proposed to before the night is out.

Pros: These places are usually not very well lit!

Cons: Everything there is old and smoky, not just the alcohol.

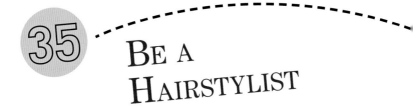

35

BE A HAIRSTYLIST

Guys have to get their hair cut all the time, and it's no treat for them when there's no barbershop to run away to.

In smaller cities and in the suburbs, sometimes there's no other choice for them than making an appointment with Debbie down at the Hair Affair. Or Tiffany at the Mane Attraction. Or Karl at Karl's Kulture Kurl.

That's when you come in (may as well be you rather than Debbie, Tiffs, or that Karl, who sounds a bit like a communist or white supremacist). As a certified cosmetologist, you can protect your poor little frightened male client from all the scary girl stuff going on around him. While you're sheltering him from talk of waxing, bleaching, and two-timing men, you'll also be bolstering his confidence. It's part of your job, anyway, so you may as well do it like you mean it. He'll go on and on about his life, you'll *hmmm* and *oooh* enthusiastically. You'll be his confidant, his better-than-best friend, because don't think for an instant that boys don't gossip. They do. And they need a shot of confidence and a sympathetic ear every four to six weeks. It's no different from what your duties will be once you've started dating, actually. Only with nicer-smelling products and better tips.

Pros: If he gets lippy, you get snippy! Put a notch in his earlobe with your super-sharp Kenchii professional shears if he gives you any 'tude.

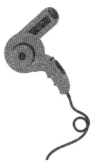

Cons: You'll have to cut hair for the very old and very young.

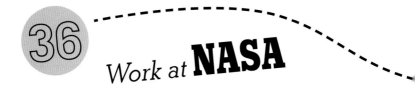

36 Work at **NASA**

You've seen The Right Stuff, Apollo 13, *and that one with the elf girl from* Lord of the Rings. Why wouldn't you want to join the exciting world of space? Not only are there loads of brilliant men who are brave and also good at math, but you'll never again have to think about what you're going to wear to work! Sure that "Space Oddity" song always freaked you out, but think about how romantic it is! "Tell my wife I love her very much . . . " You could be the one Major Tom and the boys down at ground control are talking about! You could be the one that "knoooooooooows"! You could also be the one in the spaceship hurtling out into oblivion. But it's a lot more interesting than sitting in a cubicle drinking terrible coffee every day.

Pros: No matter how out of control you get, you'll never look as bad as that crazy Depends lady.

Cons: Astronaut ice cream is SO fattening. Seriously, have you read the nutrition label?

37 Be Out **Where Major Sporting Events Are Exiting**

Be there to share in his joy or **comfort him in his sorrow.**

Either way, he'll be glad you're there. Have merchandise from both teams on hand so you can discern which way the wind is blowing and then dress accordingly. Just be careful not to look like a hooker. They like to be out when major sporting events are exiting, too.

Pros: You won't have to think of a thing to say!

Cons: There might be tears. His tears.

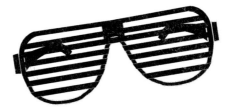

38

Go to as Many Holiday Parties as You Possibly Can

THE HOLIDAY SEASON CAN BE ESPECIALLY HARD ON A SINGLE GIRL.

There are so many functions to go to, so many chances to bring a date and show him off to your family, coworkers, or those bitches from Alpha Phi. Only you don't have a date. Another year has gone by and all you have is a great job and another promotion to show for it. We all know that that counts for nothing during Christmas party season.

So the temptation would be to stay in and watch *Emmet Otter's Jug-Band Christmas* on repeat until you've gone into a sugar coma from eating too many frosted cookies. Don't give in! Instead, go to all the parties you have to go to with your head held high and an eye on the open bar. That's where the single men congregate! And don't limit yourself to your own social functions. Crash as many others as you can! There's a much better chance that your reputation won't have preceded you at an event you weren't invited to. Find where the big investment firms are throwing their parties, or hunt down where the accountants will be ringing in the New Year. Or just hang around the nicer hotels and restaurants. Wait long enough and they will come to you.

All the couples will have the disadvantage of having to go home early because they're sensible adults and they need to go gift shopping for future in-laws in the morning. Single you, on the other hand, can stay out and spread the holiday cheer until you've found a present of your own.

Pros: The true meaning of the season: Open bars and passed appetizers as far as the eye can see!

Cons: Start dating in December, stay together for New Year's, and prepare to be dumped by Valentine's Day. Holiday party matches rarely last, so you'll have to live it up while you can. Bring an extra large handbag to take some crab cakes home with you to save for the lean months.

39

Go to Culinary School!

Culinary school is heavily male-dominated. **Grab a chef's jacket and turn up the heat.**

It's probably a good idea for you to learn how to cook, anyway. Sooner or later you'll get sick of Hamburgerless Hamburger Helper (believe it or not!) for dinner every night, and it would be nice if you had one or two other tricks in the kitchen. Pony up the cash for a class or two and see to it that you share a station with the nicest piece of meat available.

As you probably know from watching reality TV, male chefs can be scary and self-absorbed. Try to overcome your fears of being yelled at and having béarnaise sauce thrown at you. Focus on his ability to feed you. Maybe it's going to be impossible to get the red wine out of your white couch, but really, shouldn't you have known that the ten dollar bottle of merlot you got from the corner store (the corner store, of all places!) would never be fit for drinking with his beef Wellington? Honestly, woman, you have so much to learn.

Pros: Great for dinner parties! As long as he stays in the kitchen.

Cons: He'll always love the Viking range and Le Creuset crockery more than you.

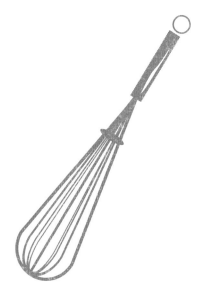

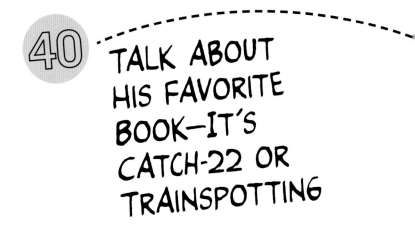

TALK ABOUT HIS FAVORITE BOOK—IT'S CATCH-22 OR TRAINSPOTTING

There are two types of men: those who have only ever read one book, and those who have read more than one book. Which is which is easy to determine. If he looks like a one-in-a-lifetime-type, don't bother talking about it—you haven't read *Gretzky: Life on the Red Line*, so don't bring it up. If, on the other hand, he looks of the more scholarly persuasion, you've got a fifty-fifty chance of correctly guessing his favorite book.

Go up to your target and say, "I loved *Trainspotting*." If this confuses him, quickly interrupt and say, "I just finished reading *Catch-22*. Wow. What a book." You'll have deftly sussed out which of the two is his Favorite Book Ever within seconds. And you'll look like the answer to his prayers. Here you are, a girl who gets him, his

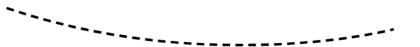

soul mate, freshly arrived from the library, ready to engage in intelligent conversation about the Most Important Book Ever Written. Run with it.

Pros: When this relationship dissolves, at least you'll have completed the reading list for the next.

Cons: There are only so many times you can use the quote "Another country heard from!" or expound upon the merits of the disgusting restaurant chapter before even you stop believing that it's sporting.

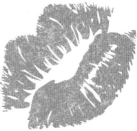

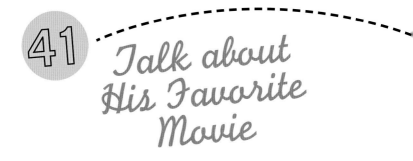

41

Talk about His Favorite Movie

There's a good possibility that his favorite movie is Terminator 2 *or The* Big Lebowski *or **The Usual Suspects.** But* it's absolutely one of those three, honestly. If not *Pulp Fiction.* Or *The Godfather.* One of those five. Definitely one of those five. When it comes to movies, there are only five types of guys. Without a doubt, no question. Watch those movies, go out, and have access to loads of men who approve of your film education and endless references they wrongly assumed you wouldn't get. Quote any of these movies and the dude will abide.

Pros: Knowing his favorite movie will explain so much. Like why he loves Pepsi; why his personal habits are disgusting; why he says, "Kevin Spacey *is* Keyser Söze" whenever you say, "I don't get it" about anything; why he loves slick, stylized, sexy violence; and why he likes to make you offers you can't refuse.

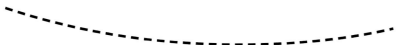

Cons: He's no film snob, so you'll have no one to go with you to the tribute to Ingmar Bergman down at the Independent Film Center.

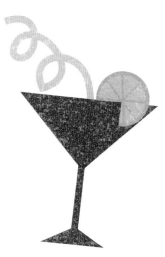

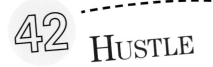

42 HUSTLE

BECOME VERY GOOD AT DARTS OR POOL.

Position yourself in a bar near the darts or the pool table. Be fascinated with the men playing darts or pool, as well as with the games themselves. When asked if you play darts or pool, open your eyes wide, shake your head vigorously, and say you've never played before in your life. Then ask if he wants to play for money. He, or one of his more adventurous friends, will instantly volunteer to teach you. You will "learn" very quickly and he will think himself a great "teacher." You will also win "all his money."

Pros: Even if you don't end up winning a man, you'll be able to put yourself through night school. Or take computer classes or something. That's almost as good, right?

Cons: Late nights of skull-numbing boredom.

PLAY POKER

43

Learn to play poker and join a regularly occurring game. **Or league.** Or match. Or whatever they call it. Aside from learning all your male opponents' secrets, you'll have a captive audience. So few women play poker, even in this age of poker popularity. One of you, five of them at the table. Millions of possible outcomes. Vegas has you going home happy at two to one.

Pros: Lots and lots of money to be made, and you can wear sunglasses the whole time.

Cons: You could lose everything you have, including the deed to your house.

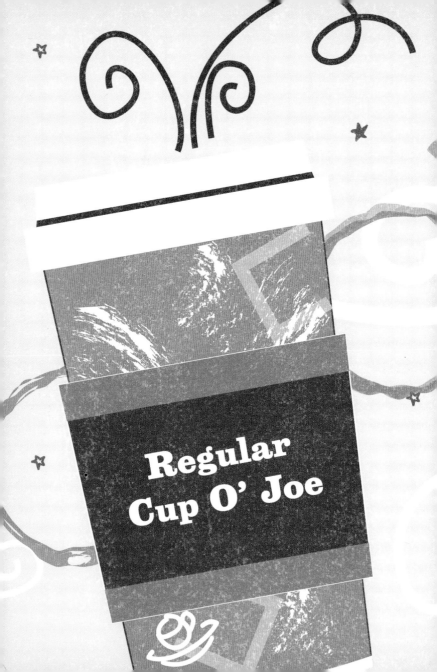

Regular
Cup O' Joe

PART THREE

SETTLE

THERE'RE WORSE THINGS.
LIKE HAVING TO GO TO YOUR
FAMILY REUNION AND REPORT
THAT YOU'RE STILL SINGLE.

ALL SALES ARE FINAL///NO REFUNDS OR RETURNS///
AVERAGE JOE CAFE///

Reconnect with the Guy You Were Too Good for in High School

Oh, how the years can humble a girl.
There you are, sitting in your studio apartment, a bottle of sauvignon blanc and a brick of brie into the evening, watching censored *Sex and the City* because that's all TBS broadcasts anymore, and—let's face it—you can't afford cable anyhow. Somewhere between ordering Chinese and switching to hard liquor, you get to wondering: whatever happened to Aaron Vandenlandenberg? He worshiped the ground you walked on back in high school. Lots of guys did. But you thought you were too good for all of them, didn't you?

And look where that's gotten you: another night alone with the bottle and television. But all is not lost. You can be that confident (albeit completely self-absorbed) girl again! With no more than a couple of clicks on Facebook, you can get the old fan club back together. Deliver some pretend

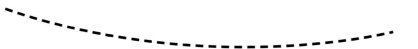

heartfelt apologies, insist you've changed/matured/
are different now, and ta-da: it's just like 1998 . . .
Forever.

Pick the most promising among them and
mention to him that you'll be back in town for
Thanksgiving. Perhaps he'd like to go to that coffee
place you and all the popular kids used to frequent?

Pros: In just a few easy steps, you've made all
his adolescent dreams come true. And you've got
yourself a lifetime of adoration.

Cons: You'll have to move back
to Chippewa Falls.

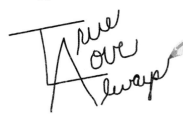

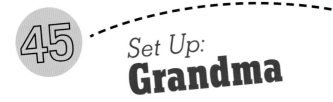

45

Set Up: Grandma

Don't think for a minute that there wasn't a time when grandma was **similarly on the prowl.** And she did it without Facebook stalking or drunken text messages, so for eff's sake: show Nana some respect.

True, she had the benefit of World War II (explaining all those letters she's kept containing marriage proposals and exotic postmarks), but she's on your side now. She's almost as ashamed as you are that you're still single. You think it's fun for her to hear about Beulah's granddaughter's wedding for the billionth time? How Beulah got a peony and orange blossom corsage and a place of honor in the front row of the church? Heck no! She is tired of being the laughingstock at bridge, so she's going to use her skills and you're going to use yours.

So if she says to go to a Bible college, by gum, you do that, missy. If she thinks that JCPenney ensemble suits you, suit up. And if she points out that men like a clean house and homemade cookies, honey, you get in that kitchen and you damn well

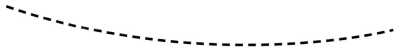

make sure it sparkles. The how and why of a man gaining access to your kitchen? Well, she's got that covered. No self-respecting, church-going young man will deny a snowy-haired old lady her request that he meet her granddaughter.

Pros: Suck it, Beulah. Street cred for both you and Grandma for as long as the relationship lasts.

Cons: Grandma's beginning to not see so well anymore. . . . She probably had no idea that the bowling shoe attendant is pushing sixty.

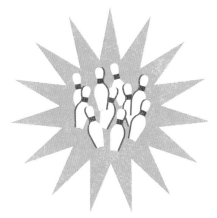

46 SET UP: YOUR MOM MUST KNOW SOMEONE

Mom loves you no matter what. Unlike Grandma, she doesn't care if you have a boyfriend, **as long as you're happy.** But wouldn't it be nice if for once you could go visit her and have someone else do all the heavy-lifting projects that Mom can't do by herself? You're up to the challenge now, but even you know your days of spryly retrieving the artificial Christmas tree from the basement are numbered. Likewise, rearranging the living room furniture. And same goes for flipping the mattresses. Best to see if Mom can't come up with someone else besides her devoted daughter for those tasks. And even better if that guy can be the same person who does your tree retrieval, rearranging, and flipping. This is, hopefully, what she'll keep in mind when looking for a suitable mate for you. Sure she knows you deserve Prince Charming, but she'll be smart enough to look out for Prince Here. So give her your parameters (anyone, Mom, anyone . . . I'm so tired of yard work . . . so very tired) and take what she can get.

Pros: At least your mom likes him! I can hear her wedding toast already.

Cons: Mom has a track record of finding the youngest, most inexperienced guy for the job. Remember the fourteen-year-olds she got to paint the house? And the barely legal kid who refinished the floors? You'll have to—wait—no, never mind. That's not a con at all. Go on, you cougar, you.

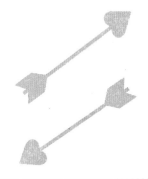

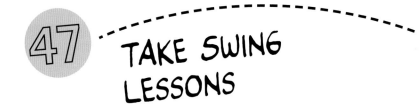

47

TAKE SWING LESSONS

Remember 1998? The year that Gap commercial debuted? The one that launched the new golden age of swing? All of a sudden everyone's favorite movies were *Swing Kids* and *Swingers*, and there was nothing more fun than going down to the VFW to jitterbug with your friends and some old people who would teach you how to do it. You did your hair all fancy and bought circle skirts and t-strap heels. And the boys were nice to you because they had to be. It was all part of the game. But then school started again and you had to leave your seamed stockings behind.

Well, curiously enough, for some guys, the cultural revolution that saw the permanent retirement of your Big Bad Voodoo Daddy CDs never happened! Like how the Renaissance never made it to Russia, or the Dark Ages to the Middle East, there are still some men out there fox-trotting and jiving as if it were still cool to wear a white T-shirt and khakis. Find them and you'll have yourself someone to make you look good on every dance floor for the rest of your life.

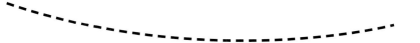

Pros: Twirling! And applause!

Cons: He's a geek with a fedora and loafers. You wouldn't want to take him anywhere where there isn't a 90 percent chance they'll be playing "Sing, Sing, Sing."

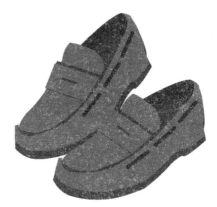

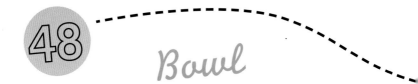

48

Bowl

Not everyone had a bowling unit in gym class during high school.

Pity, because the girl who can kegel will definitely score well with a certain set of men. **And she'll have them all to herself.**

Bowling is easy. Just line up the ball with the pins and you're pretty much set. But if for some reason it isn't working for you, there will be plenty of men in your group or in the next lane willing to show you how it's done. If you're naturally good at it, all the better. You'll be the MVP and a girl. Imagine that! You are a keeper indeed.

Pros: It's the only sport where you can drink and eat while playing it! Get another pitcher of beer and order another pizza.

Cons: Blink and all of a sudden you've acquired the portly, pasty physique of a professional bowler.

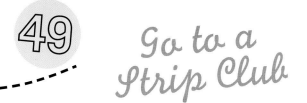

49 Go to a Strip Club

Guys say this works because it shows what a cool girl you are.

This presupposes, of course, that their definition of cool is the **willingness to blatantly objectify other women.** So, sure, if you don't mind betraying the generations of women who came before you and fought for the near equality you enjoy today, go for it! Maybe some of those singles you stick in that girl's G-string will be put toward her PhD in economics. You never know.

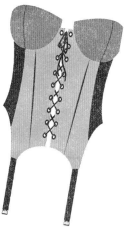

Pros: Strip clubs are the one place in the world where there's a shorter line to the ladies' room than there is for the men's!

Cons: Blatantly objectifying other women.

BE THE STOP SIGN GIRL AT A CONSTRUCTION SITE

What better way to get noticed than by being the girl who holds the stop/slow sign at a highway construction site? Standing in the middle of the road for eight to ten hours a day, telling motorists when it's safe for them to use the one open lane of traffic will certainly display you to fine advantage—assuming you can pull off a high-visibility reflector vest and hardhat. If they're not all rolling down their windows asking for your number, then they are too dense to know what they're missing. You'll have to settle for one of the guys on your crew. Which is by no means truly settling, since when's the last time you dated a guy who

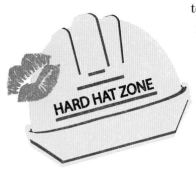

HARD HAT ZONE

didn't think a backhoe was something dirty and, moreover, could operate one?

Not every girl with this gig is super connected. You don't need a brother in the crew or a dad who owns the company. All you need is the yellow pages. The second you pull up to their offices, they'll be falling over themselves to get you equipped and out on the road.

Pros: A great tan!

Cons: Skin cancer!

51

BECOME A GROUPIE FOR A LOCAL BAND

This isn't quite as psychologically draining as adopting an artist (see #80), nor is it as tedious as hanging out with the hipsters at twee indie pop rock concerts (see #82). Even so, it's best to try to like the band and to have earplugs on hand.

It's easy to become a groupie when you're dealing with local-band level of talent. They probably don't have very many of you! You'll be noticed immediately, so try to pick the band with the fewest attractive women fans and hottest tech guys, manager, and musicians. From there, it's just a matter of showing up night after ear-splitting night and showing your commitment.

Men never love attention as much as they love their first attention, so whether you're fawning over the lead singer, manager, sound guy, or tyro journalist trying to put together a fan 'zine devoted to this, the next big thing, you'll be adored for your good taste

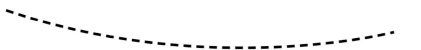

and have a special place in all their hearts as well as in the van after the gig.

Pros: He'll look back on his band days, remember your devotion, and think maybe he could have made it. Aw.

Cons: He'll look back on band days, remember your devotion, and think maybe he could have made it. Shudder.

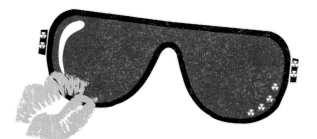

52

Wear a **Claddagh Ring**

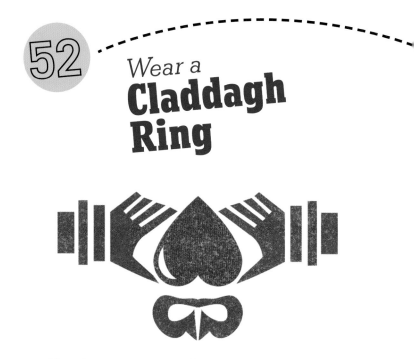

Has it ever occurred to you that maybe you're not being asked out because guys assume you're already taken? Because a charming thing like yourself is too great a catch to be single? No? That hasn't ever occurred to you? Not once? Well, sit back and dream a little.

Heaven knows what goes on in those heads of theirs, but smart money says it's a confusing and dark place. Best to make negotiating the You situation as easy as possible for them. That's why you need a Claddagh ring, those awful Irish rings with the heart and the hands and the crown and all the other symbols that the Galwegian fishermen could think of back in seventeenth-century Ireland to denote love and friendship and fealty.

Yes, it'd be nice if you didn't have to buy one for yourself. It's true there aren't a lot of things more depressing than buying your own damn ring, but this one is an investment. Get one, wear it with the heart pointing out to denote your unbelievable single status, and see what comes your way. At least it'll be more than you had before. And you got a piece of jewelry out of the deal. Such as it is.

Pros: You won't have to do anything overtly embarrassing to advertise that you're single, like ride around alone on a tandem bicycle or have an unevenly distributed fake tan because you don't have anyone to do the places you can't reach.

Cons: This will most likely attract the Irish, men of Irish decent, or guys from Boston. Consider yourself warned.

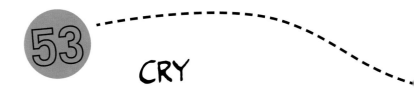

53

CRY

Men do not know what to do with a woman who is crying. **They have two reactions.** One is to immediately try to soothe you by being super nice. Start crying in front of the right guy and he will give you the world if it will make your sobbing cease.

Pros: Finally, commitment! He said he wants to take you out sometime/thinks you should be more than friends/loves you! There now, don't you feel better?

Cons: There's a fifty-fifty chance it will work. If he's not the placating type, you're in trouble. (See #54.)

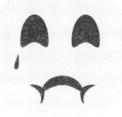

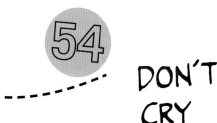

DON'T CRY

The other reaction guys have to a crying woman is disgust and repulsion. **And the administering of something to cry about.** That's bad news. So, suck it up and save the crying for when he's out of earshot. Of course, still tell him all about the terrible thing that happened to you. He will admire how you're not crying. How great it is that you're so stoical and that you keep all your real feelings to yourself. That's a load off him!

Pros: He's less afraid of giving it a shot with a woman who won't be crying all the time.

Cons: You're about to date a sociopath!

55

Be a Hired Girl on a Farm

There might not be too many opportunities for this, now that we don't all live off the land, but if you can get yourself a position as a hired girl, you're sitting pretty.

Your parents probably have enough of a workforce on their own farm, thanks to all your brothers and sisters, so it might be a good time for you to go seek your fortune.

Find a neighboring farm in search of a little domestic help. Be careful to select one with married daughters and one unmarried son. Soon the mother will fall in love with you because you're so clean and efficient. And you make such good bread! The father will love your ability to iron shirts. In just a few short weeks or months, they will see you as the only solution to the problem of their unmarried son.

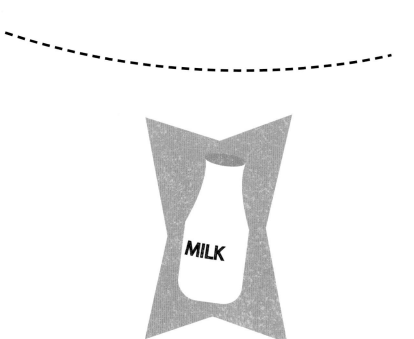

Congratulations! You took a simple live-in, round-the-clock, hard-labor job and turned it into the exact same thing, only now with a husband to look after!

Pros: When his parents kick the bucket, you get the farm!

Cons: You get the farm!

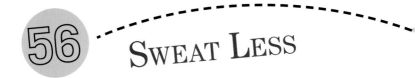

56 SWEAT LESS

No matter how pretty and smart and funny you are, sweating too much is going to be a deal breaker. **It's very** distracting for a guy when you're chatting him up at a bar or a barbeque or a baptism and you're "glowing" just a little too much.

Some women, like some men, perspire too much. They can't help it. If someone tells them, "Oh, hey, you're sweating a lot," they're not able to do anything about it except sweat more, having been hugely embarrassed by someone pointing it out.

For men, it's not such a big deal. Men are supposed to sweat, and it's assumed that they were recently doing something manly, like moving a couch. But you? You've got no excuse. It's a terrible affliction, and if you've got it, you need to strategize.

Start by going to the bathroom a lot and running your wrists and elbows under cold water. If that doesn't cool you down, find the darkest corner and hide there with an ice water until your body temperature has regained control of itself. If it's still not helping, go home and wait until there's a cure for your problem.

Only attend events that are well air-conditioned and dark. And ones where you don't have to do too much physical activity like climb steps or stand. It'll cut down on your chances at finding a boyfriend, yes, but you'll have a much better shot at making the chances you do have worth it because you won't be known as that weird sweaty girl.

Pros: By dropping off the face of the social planet, you'll make yourself exclusive and sought-after!

Cons: You might end up never leaving the basement.

57

Hit Up **the** **County Fairs** (and the Carnies)

There's nothing quite as alluring as the smell of deep-fried sugar mingling with the smell of the livestock pavilion. County fairs are an amazing store of delicious food, adorable animals, challenging games, and rides for every age, shape, and size.

Even if all you care to do is show up, you can't go wrong. There'll be strapping young guys, in from the farm, gearing up for the tractor pull! Carnies with their quaint little ways, spewing racist phrases you haven't heard since great-uncle Bill died! And if you really want to be in control of the situation and get the attention you deserve, become part of the action. Be the weight guesser! Or raise prize Holsteins! Put yourself out there for all the eligible men in the county, as well as your new carnie friends, and there's every reason to believe you'll be going home a grand champion.

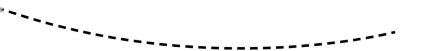

Pros: If all else fails, you can ride the Bullet until you throw up all the cotton candy and funnel cake you've been gorging on. That'll get you noticed.

Cons: You don't know what all those scary farm animals eat. What if they have a taste for scrappy girls looking for boyfriends? You can almost see it in their eyes. *Run!*

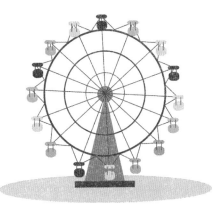

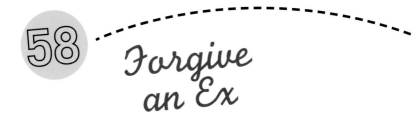

58

Forgive an Ex

It seemed like a good idea at the time, having a zero-tolerance policy for guys who cheated on you, thought about **cheating on you, jokingly threatened to cheat on you, or in any other way annoyed you.** It certainly was empowering to storm out of all those relationships with all that righteous fury and it was absolutely gratifying to tell everyone about it. The story of how you shoved the dozen roses he sent in a Jiffy Mailer and FedExed them back to him is one for the ages. But as satisfying as that was, your high standards and big deal morals have earned you naught but another night eating alone over the kitchen sink.

Maybe it's time to stable your high horse and remember the good parts about your wayward exes. Sure it was traumatic the time you went over to his house and found that used pregnancy test (and honestly, who keeps those things?), but he was so good at computers! So what if he drunkenly dragged you through that field resulting in the most horrific sprained ankle that you then had to walk home on because he was sure a cab would take too long to arrive. Remember how you loved his mom?

Anyway, that's all in the past. As were your exes' silly transgressions. Look one up, graciously forgive him, and live resigned-to-your-fate ever after.

Pros: You know what you're getting into.

Cons: You will look like a fool in front of all your friends who were so supportive of your decision to get rid of the creep.

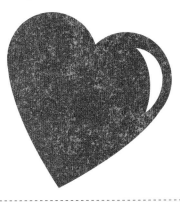

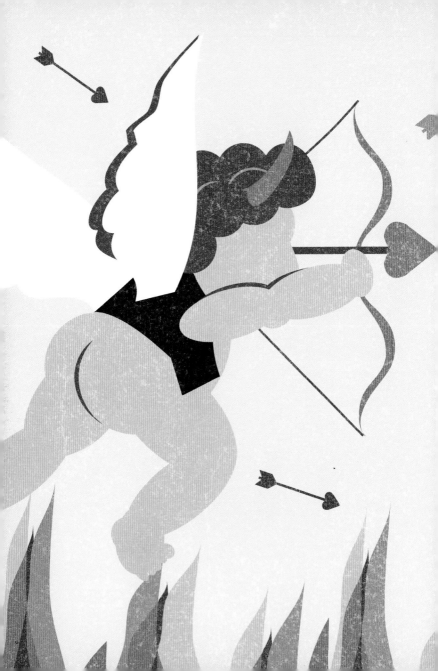

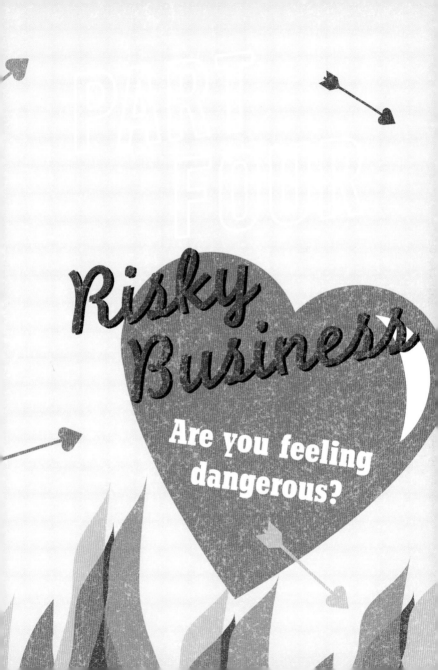

Risky Business

Are you feeling dangerous?

59 DIP YOUR PEN IN COMPANY INK

This is not for the faint of heart. Nor is it for the very young or the loose-lipped. And if you just started your job, or are the intern, don't even think about it. But an established woman can pull this off with the same élan she uses to close high-powered deals. If you're smart about it, marvelously inappropriate good times are just a workday away.

Your task is simple: No more of that "I don't care if I haven't washed my hair in two days, it's only work" mentality. And for crying out loud, would it kill you to maintain your lip gloss? Yes, it comes right off every time you refill on coffee, but this is more important than convenience or consumption of cosmetics not entirely fit for human ingestion. Once you've bothered to keep yourself up for a couple of weeks, make your move.

And by move, I mean find every reason to stop by his office or email him. You can't rush these

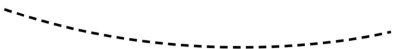

things, but believe me, if you play your cards right, you'll have something much more appealing than the karaoke bar to look forward to for entertainment after the company Christmas party.

Pros: You've never looked better! You're going to work on time! Your career will take off thanks to your new dedication!

Cons: Everyone knows about it. Everyone.

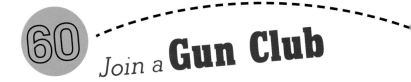

60 Join a **Gun Club**

What's more attractive than a cute young thing like yourself knowing what kind of gun James Bond uses? Or how to load a Glock? Or what the term "open sights" means? Absolutely nothing.

Now you're probably thinking: it's one thing to be able to use your gun knowledge to impress a Republican at a dinner party, and another to pull the trigger. But to really be on target for a lasting relationship, a gun club is the way to go. If you're not from the South or Midwest, or you don't have fathers, brothers, or male cousins, you're best off looking up your local gun club online or in the yellow pages.

This won't work very well if you actually look like a wilderness-type. The more feminine you are, the more surprising and adorable your tales of practicing out at the lake with body targets will be. So be sure to mention your skills while wearing lots of pink, applying lip gloss, driving a Mazda Miata, or sipping a Malibu and Diet.

You'll also have to check your local laws (it won't surprise you to learn that it's more difficult to get a gun—legally—in New York City than Little Falls, Minnesota), but believe it or not, it's pretty easy to buy and register a little .22 rifle and start practicing down at the club. Most clubs have fees, and bullets (or "ammo," or "shells," as you will call them) can be pretty pricey, but all told, it's an investment. You will be the only woman there and have your pick of all the intrigued men.

Pros: The power to kill.

Cons: The power to kill . . . accidentally. All you're trying to do is get a boyfriend, not be some sort of vigilante superhero. Maybe you're not ready for a gun. Consider bow hunting?

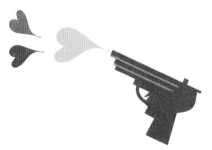

61

Join the Armed Forces (or Work on Base)

This is especially good for young ladies who aren't wild about commitment.

Whether you're enlisted or simply work at the base's laundromat, the selection is endless. And they're all in such good shape. And you will be too. All those drills, all those impossible acts of derring-do, all that pushing yourself to the limit . . . and that's not necessarily because you're actually in the army.

Pros: You're finally giving back to your country . . . even if you never see combat.

Cons: You'll end up giving more to them than they give back. There's no Purple Heart for generous girlfriend-ry.

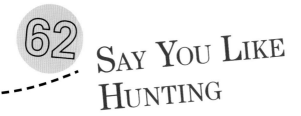

62 SAY YOU LIKE HUNTING

Not all men are metrosexuals, hipsters, or gay. Remember the luck you had when you told that guy about passing the test for your concealed weapons permit? There're some who will be equally turned on when you say you like hunting, and wax lyrical about waking up early on those crisp fall mornings, pulling on your camo and blaze-orange over your long underwear, dousing yourself with doe urine, loading your 30-30 Marlin lever action, and having at the local deer population. How poetic. There's nothing like experiencing the majesty of the wilderness and getting more in touch with God's magnificent creation to make a girl want to go blast something's head off.

Pros: You'll need to know all this anyway if you're ever running for senate in Minnesota.

Cons: Again, the power to kill . . . accidentally. You didn't learn your lesson with the guns? Oh my gosh, look! You killed Bambi's mom. And what's that over there? Oh man, Bambi, too.

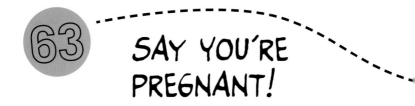

63 SAY YOU'RE PREGNANT!

Though some might say this borders less on cute and more on crazy, **pretending to be pregnant is at best *Knocked Up* and at worst** *Fatal Attraction.* Watch both before you continue.

As probably one of the most despicable things you can do to a man, and really more for if you want a husband, this last resort move is a guaranteed man-lander if you can pull it off. If you can't, however, you'd best consider this relationship a "restraining order" and move on to a less clever chap.

Note: It's best to say you *think* you're pregnant, unless you're a Juilliard grad with a practiced miscarriage monologue, or you're actually pregnant.

Pros: You've read *Jude the Obscure.* 'Nuff said.

Cons: Your likelihood of being booed on the Maury Povich show rises exponentially.

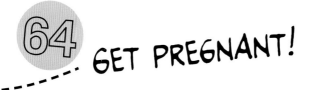

64 GET PREGNANT!

This is a fun task with no long-term consequences. Ask anyone.

Pros: You get to name it and dress it and everything!

Cons: What cons? Flush those pills, sister.

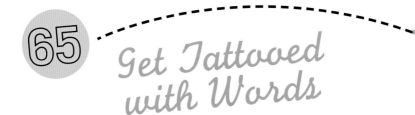

65 Get Tattooed with Words

Do you know why that one girl you know is adored by men?

Not because she knows a lot about music or can shotgun a pint of Guinness, but because she happens to have the first stanza of *The Waste Land* tattooed at the base of her neck. Men flock to her in droves because she's got an easy conversation starter printed right there for all to see. She is a magnet for frat boys, goth boys, farmers, factory workers, scholars, and anyone else who happens to be male. When she feels like being left alone, she wears turtlenecks or polo shirts, but where's the fun in that? Wherever she walks, there's a trail of interested men in her wake.

A tattoo is a big commitment, but if you're considering getting one, there's no more bang for your buck than getting one that's text-heavy. You won't be able to move for all the men tapping you on your shoulder and asking if they can read what's on your back. All you have to do is decide which ones will get to. And be sure to have a short lesson prepared in the event that they are unfamiliar with the quoted work. See? They'll find out how smart you are too!

Pros: That part in *Anna Karenina* is so beautiful. Now you get to share it with a larger audience!

Cons: You thought you loved Tolstoy. Then you learned that he all but abandoned his family when he decided to renounce his wealth and live like a peasant. Maybe not such a swell guy after all. How are you going to reconcile your feminist principles with what's tattooed on your forearm?

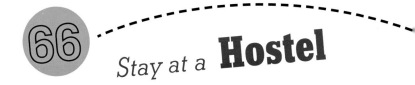

Stay at a **Hostel**

Deep breath. In, out, good. Yes, there're lots of smelly people. That's normal. **And lots of giant backpacks.** That's to be expected too. And yes, everyone around you thinks he or she is superior to you because he or she's seen the real Europe. They all smoke rollies and drink the local pilsner, not because those things are cheaper than Camels or whiskey (though they are), but because they are more *authentic* and therefore better than anything your cake-eating-princess self knows anything about.

If you can get over their unwashed pretentiousness, you're nearly there. So now, suck it up and reserve a bed in one of the dormitories. Yes, there will be gross men sleeping naked on top of the sheets. You just have to put that out of your mind. Focus on finding your new, idealistic, tragically out-of-touch boyfriend. Drink a bottle of your favorite imperialist, capitalist, or aspirational wine to take the edge off. Careful not to let anyone see. Then—no, it's not going to be pleasant, but bite the bullet—find a group in the common free Wi-Fi area, produce a deck of cards, and ask if anyone wants to play "President A-hole" or "Petty Bourgeois Pig" or "Mao" or any other combination of words that might be the name of a card game that these smelly hippies seem to enjoy on trains or in moldy rooms when they should be out seeing the sights. Only they can't afford to see the sights because they've never actually worked a day in their privileged lives, because to do so would be admitting that they're mainstream, when really they're not because they are going to buck the system and go travel, Dad, because just because you went to college and met Mom and moved to suburbia doesn't mean I have to, okay?

Pros: Chances are he's sitting on a trust fund back in Connecticut.

Cons: Chances are you'll be catching more than a man . . . Just look at that shower floor. And those mattresses. And the kitchen area. And everyone else's hair . . .

67 LOITER AT A JEWELRY STORE

Or work there. Whatever's the easiest way for you to target idealistic men shopping for engagement rings. If you're behind the counter or if you're just "browsing" close by, gush with all the insincerity in the world and ask what the lucky girl's name is. And then say "Oh Diana? Diana *Fluffnufferton*? Um, sure. Yeah, that's . . . great . . . it's just that . . . well, I probably shouldn't say but . . . she's been in here before. . . . She's been a lot of places before" and proceed with demolishing her reputation! He'll be crushed to find out whatever you just said about his fiancée, and you'll be a shoulder to cry on.

Or, if you're working in the fancy watch department (which, other than the fancy engagement ring department, should be the only reason an unmarried man needs ever set foot in a jewelry store), you can wind your way into his heart with much less maliciousness. But where's the fun in that?

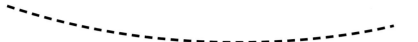

Pros: You can get him a discount on your engagement ring, or at the very least, he'll know what you like.

Cons: All those smug women who come in with their fiancés. They think they're so great.

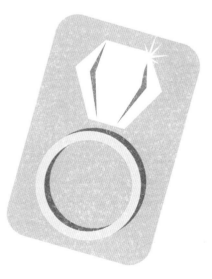

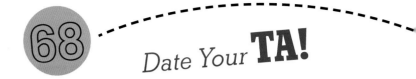

68

Date Your **TA!**

Let there be no misunderstanding: enrolling yourself in an institution of higher education, spending all of the **fall semester looking for a guy and then letting one get you pregnant definitely works.** But sooner or later, you're going to get called into a concerned educator's office and asked if you're in school to get a degree or to get a man. Ouch! And wouldn't you want someone who has already graduated and has a job? And for those reasons, you should get your eyes off your classmates, and pay attention to the teacher, for once. In fact, preemptively date the concerned educator, who is most likely your TA, that adorable PhD candidate who is in charge of teaching you because the professor is too busy writing journal articles to do it himself.

First things first: you need to be enrolled in a school. It doesn't have to be a really good one, but you need some class to attend. Second, you have to be either amazing or bad at it. He's never going to notice you if you're average. Either strategy comes with its own set of challenges, so just go with what comes naturally. There's plenty of unnatural stuff ahead of you, so spare yourself while you can.

At some point (preferably early on) in the semester, you're going to have to go to his office to discuss either your failing grades or your brilliantly conceived twenty page essay on how the laws of thermodynamics apply to last year's Oscar attire. Once you've perched yourself on the folding chair in his third of the basement office, all you have to do is turn on the charm. Talk about something other than his class. He'll never see that coming! And he'll never have guessed that you had such intelligent/stupid things to say! This will require further discussion, either over coffee in the Quad or at the fancy grad school bar downtown. Once you're there, you're in. Say hello to Mrs. Professor Whatever.

Pros: He's so smart! So eccentric. So fascinating-but-also-alienating at dinner parties. And you get to be the adorable young thing on his brilliant arm.

Cons: If he did it once, he'll probably do it again. After all, once your adorable factor wears out, he'll want another one.

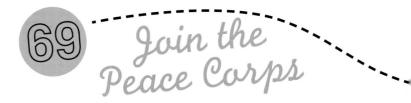

69 Join the Peace Corps

If learning a new language and immersing yourself in a developing world's culture for two years doesn't **prove your commitment to finding a boyfriend, then nothing will.** And it's not like you were doing anything more productive with your time now, were you?

More men than women join the Peace Corps, so you've already got the advantage over all your friends who are trying online dating. What's up now, Kimmy? She'll be dying of jealousy while you're having the last laugh in . . . um, Eritrea, wherever that is. And then, think of all the grateful and gorgeous locals, dying to be with your benevolent, English-teaching, ditch-digging, vaccine-administering, clean water–supplying self because you represent all that is good in the world. Or something like that, anyway.

Pros: You might end up in a place like Liberia or Rwanda, where women have more representation in government than they do in the United States! You could bring back so much more than a man when your stint is over.

Cons: Not everyone comes back.

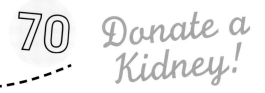

70 Donate a Kidney!

Donate a kidney to a guy and you're set. Dude will owe you big time and the least he can do is be a devoted mate for **the rest of his dialysis-free life.** And no matter what, there's no argument that can't be won with your trump card: "Oh my gosh, I cannot believe you just said/did/thought that. You are alive because of me. I gave you a kidney, you jerk."

Pros: You'll always be a part of him. And if he dumps you, you can sue him for the black market value of your kidney, which, at press time, was about $11,000. Not bad!

Cons: You might need your spare later. Then you'll be stuck getting another from some opportunist creep who will forever lord his generosity over you. What a pain.

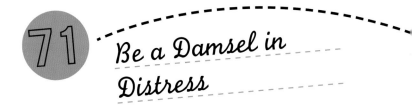

Be a Damsel in Distress

There's nothing like seeing an attractive woman on the side of the road with a **flat tire to bring out the chivalry in a man.** In fact, that might be the only thing.

The side of any random road is kind of risky, though. Who knows what the universe will send you? Better off having problems directly in front of your apartment where, if need be, you can go right up to the door of that mysterious bachelor and ask for help. Or at the parking lot at work when the sales guys are leaving for the day. Or the parking lot of the Green Bay Packers practice facility. Go on. It's worth a shot.

If fate needs a little push and you have to bring a penknife to do the damage yourself, so be it. It's only a tire. And you've got AAA. No big deal.

Once your gallant savior has fixed you up, be sure to find out where to bring thank you cookies the next day. The cookies part is key. The whole operation goes down the tubes if you fail to deliver cookies. And nothing too fancy either—stick with

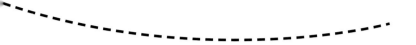

traditional chocolate chip, or oatmeal raisin if you're feeling wild. Once traditional gender roles are established, you'll be off Single Street and merging onto Happy Couple Highway.

Pros: Someone to come to your rescue for the rest of your life! Or at least the next five to ten years.

Cons: That cookies trick you pulled established a dangerous precedent. Now he's conditioned, so be ready to be in the kitchen every time he's done something decent for you.

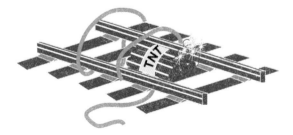

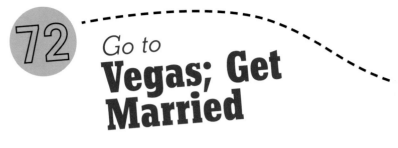

72

Go to Vegas; Get Married

Okay, so quickie Vegas marriages brought on by drinking beverages measured out in yards are seldom the **kind of thing you'll end up telling the grandkids about.** But it *is* a good bonding experience. Think about all the opportunities you'll have to get to know each other—to let your marriage blossom into love—as you work together to get a quickie Reno divorce. You'll need to confirm his social security number and he'll need to find out your last name, there will be frantic faxes back and forth with bank information and signatures. There's no truer test of character than having to do paperwork, and once you've seen each other shine under those circumstances, you both might reconsider going through the hassle of having to find a notary.

Pros: No need to move! You can have one of those glamorous "open marriages" where you get to keep your independence!

Cons: The wedding album.

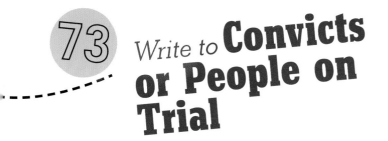

73 *Write to* **Convicts or People on Trial**

You're lonely, they're lonely, let love defy the prison walls. **So he stole Trevelyan's corn so the young might see the morn.** Or he shot a man in Reno, just to watch him die. Or maybe he made the ill-advised decision to fight the law. And the law won.

Great relationships can come from letter writing (see #2), and you'll be adored even more if you write to a guy in jail with nothing better to do and lots of time to think about you. Another great choice is to find a guy who hasn't yet been sent up the river but stands a pretty good chance of it, depending whether or not the jury swallows his testimony. Start writing to him and you'll be the brave girl who stood by him, even up to and through his incarceration. And if for some reason he's not guilty, you'll have a date for after the trial.

Pros: You know he won't cheat on you—with a girl, anyway.

Cons: He'll cheat on you—and not with a girl.

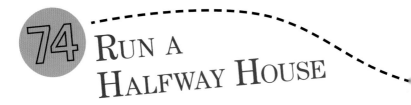

74 RUN A HALFWAY HOUSE

Help broken men find their potential as rehabilitated citizens of the world and **your possible boyfriend.**

What a satisfying feeling it will be to know you're responsible for so many brave souls just trying to make it back to mainstream society. You'll cook for them, clean for them, keep them from hurting one another, and make sure they're going to the job interviews you've lined up for them. It won't be much different from your last boyfriend, will it?

Pros: You'll save so much money on tattoos and gym equipment because Bowzer here knows how to use charcoal and a shank to do his ink at home, and he can make anything into a pull-up bar.

Cons: Relapse. Horrible, bloody, carnage-filled relapse.

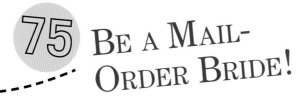

75 BE A MAIL-ORDER BRIDE!

You've been sent for! That's so exciting!
And he's paid for your train ticket and everything?
How romantic! Get ready for the adventure of a lifetime!

Now of course you must be thinking, "What kind of woman agrees to marry some guy she's never even seen? He's probably a creepy old pervert. This is a terrible idea." Well, hang on there, missy! That kind of attitude will never prevail, and who's the single one here, anyway, hmmm? That's right. Now listen: Who's ever heard of a mail-order bride actually marrying the guy she's traveling to meet? Right? She never makes it to Prospector's Cove or wherever because invariably she meets some guy on the train, or her fiancé's cuter, younger friend. So you see, this is not such a crazy idea after all.

Pros: You get to see the world!

Cons: Wife stealing is a hanging offense. You and your dashing abductor better be ready to run.

76

Befriend the Local Foreign Population!

THEY'RE FRESH OFF THE BOAT AND HAVE NO IDEA YOU'RE NOT THE BEST THEY CAN GET. STRIKE WHILE THE SAMOVAR IS HOT.

Every city has areas where the immigrants go when they've first moved to the country. Just follow the smell of authentic ethnic cuisine or the sound of ethnic music, and you'll find a vast array of new boyfriends with interesting accents.

Your new foreign male friends will be so grateful that a street-smart woman like yourself has chosen to take them under her wing. What a country! You can show them how to perform essential day-to-day tasks such as "driving a car," "ordering food for delivery," and "living a life free of religious or political persecution." They will love you for it! What's more, they'll become increasingly dependent on you! They couldn't imagine a life here in this wonderful country without you. They will spend hours painting portraits of your beautiful face. That's why one of them is going to be dating you at all times, or least until they've become naturalized citizens.

Pros: Getting to say, "No, in my country, it's a grave insult to any single girl if you make her pay for anything. Civil wars have been waged for less than the price of a pack of gum."

Cons: *Not Without My Daughter.* Watch that movie before you go back to the home country.

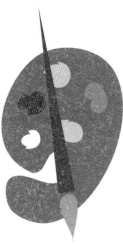

77

BE THE LOCAL FOREIGN POPULATION

Aw, look at her! With her cute accent and complete inability to speak our language. **Oh look! She doesn't even know how to use the public transportation system in our country.** She's getting all frustrated and stomping her foot and now she's talking really loudly because she thinks it will help us understand. And she has no idea how much money she just dropped. Just because it's coins doesn't mean it's not worth a whole lot more than your paper money, love! Ha ha ha.

Men in your new adopted country will love you. Just don't be too flashy and try to make a real effort to understand their culture. You don't need to sew Canadian flags on everything you own; they'll find out who you are soon enough. Even if you've moved to a country full of supermodels (avoid Scandinavia, anyway—it gets so cold and dark!), men will be attracted to you because you are different. Even if it's different in a bad way, they won't notice. They'll only

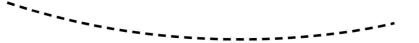

register that something about you isn't the same as other girls they know. Then they'll be queuing up to teach you simple day-to-day tasks, like "making your own food because there's no delivery," "driving a tiny, cheaply-made manual transmission car on the wrong side of the road," and "living a life in the specter of religious and political persecution." And the best part for them is that you won't know they're not the best you can get!

Pros: Learning the interesting little customs of your new country. Who knew it's tradition for the foreign girl to pay for the first, third, and last round of drinks? As well as every packet of weird potato chips that anyone in your party wants. Different cultures are so fascinating!

Cons: He's probably just looking for a Green Card and will disappear the second you've moved back home and gotten married.

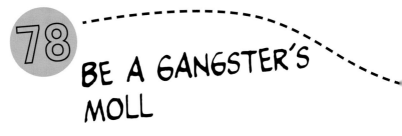

78 BE A GANGSTER'S MOLL

Obviously, he's just using you for your smarts, smoldering good looks, **nonchalant attitude toward** him and this whole messy gangstering business, and how cool you are under pressure, but that doesn't mean his cronies, enemies, or those Feds who are trailing you aren't all looking at you with an eye for something more. They've seen the goods. Now they all want you for themselves.

Pros: How empowering! And you get to wear hats and dark red lipstick.

Cons: Once you've committed to the accessory of your choice, you'll have to disappear before the boss catches on, or else he'll make you disappear. In a more permanent way than legging it to Argentina.

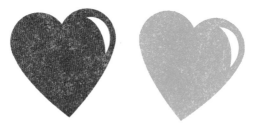

79 GET HIT BY A PUCK OR A FOUL BALL

There are still gentlemen in this world, including professional athletes contractually obligated **to visit a person in the hospital after they've put her there.**

A moment of incredible blinding pain for you, but after that, a lifetime of love. Here's your chance to land hunky pro athlete. Getting hit in the head by a frozen hockey puck or a baseball traveling at 110 miles per hour guarantees you a trip to the ER and a chat with the guy whose deflected slapshot or foul ball landed you there. The visit will have to wait until after the game at least, or more likely the next day, so you can't bounce back too quickly from your head injury. By then you'll look so much better than his other casualties. Maybe, just maybe, this all happened for a reason.

Pros: Free tickets.

Cons: Paparazzi, permanent brain damage.

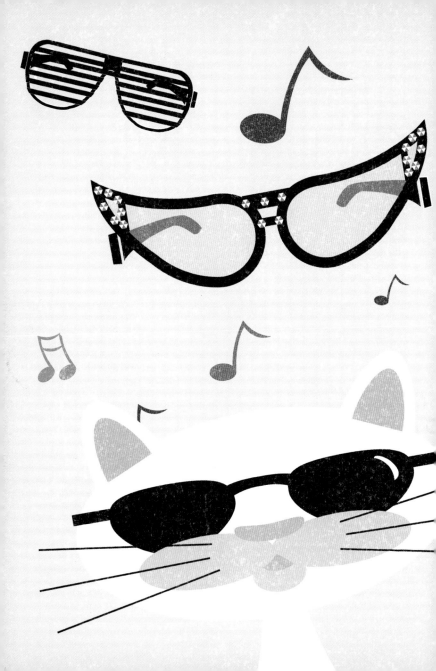

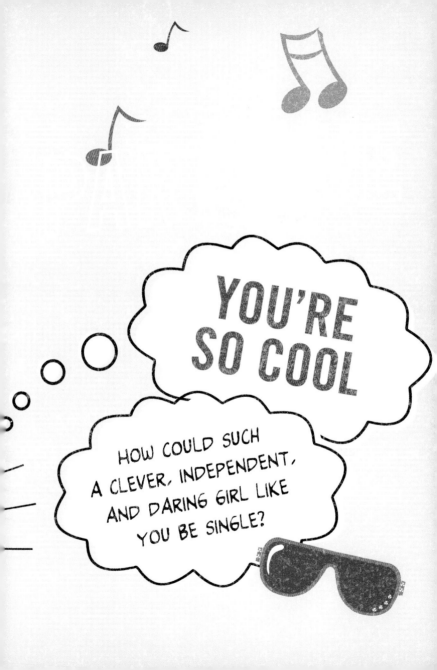

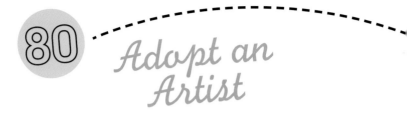

80 Adopt an Artist

Though you might not prefer the whiny, oversensitive, insecure types, **when the going gets tough,** an open mic night just might be your chance to bag the next John Mayer. Artists— whether painters, writers, actors, or musicians—can be excellent boyfriends thanks to their dreamy good looks, questionable talent, and superb skills in the bedroom (though that may be the joint you shared in the back of the equipment van). And there are plenty of emo-hunks seeking groupies. Every girl should have an artist brooding about in the wings of her phonebook.

In addition to the above-mentioned open mic nights, artists can be found at gallery openings, readings, and your local coffee shop (both in front of and behind the counter). It's really not hard to bag one. All you have to do is ask him a question about his "art," nod enthusiastically, and talk sparingly (as if you'll have the choice!). Be sure to say nothing at all that can be construed as judgmental—even something as innocuous as "Oh, I imagine I'd prefer doing film to theater if I were an actor" can and *will* be taken with as much umbrage as if you'd said something unkind about his shirt. These are giant yet fragile egos we're working with here, ladies. Open your mouth with care.

Since your artist will, naturally, be "in between projects," don't expect nights out on the town with your new boyfriend unless you're paying for them. The upside of this is that you'll have lots of time to spend in the sack, and there's no better between the sheets than an artist.

Pros: Perfect for rebounds, flings, one-night stands.

Cons: A big responsibility. You'll be in charge of the feeding and maintenance of both him and his sense of self. Also, it's not going to work out in the long run (never does, sorry!), so brace yourself for the inevitable hit single/short story/one man play/exhibition called "My Ex-Girlfriend Is a Selfish Slut Who Only Ever Used Me for Sex."

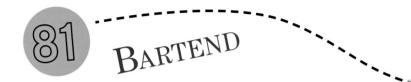

81 BARTEND

Men adore women who deliver them alcohol. **Ask any man if you can get him a beer and he will say yes.** Think all those barmaids with wedding rings are just wearing them to ward off unwanted advances? Get real. It's because they're actually married, having met great guys at their bartending job. Yep, if you're going to have to stand around all night having men talk about themselves, complain about their job, and make otherwise inane conversation, you may as well be in a bar. And what's better than being the local go-to girl for a shoulder to cry on and the administration of cure-all alcohol? Getting paid for it, that's what.

Pros: You'd probably end up there, anyway. This way your drinking problem might be curbed, or justified.

Cons: All those cash-strapped hipsters who come in after their shift at Trader Joe's, ordering, "Um, I don't know, whatever's cheapest," and leaving fifty-cent tips.

82 GO TO A BELLE AND SEBASTIAN CONCERT

Shaggy hair, striped sweaters, and square-framed glasses. Check it out! You're at a Belle and Sebastian concert. Get ready to meet a sweet and sensitive guy who will immediately think highly of you because your taste in music is as good as his. Now, you might be thinking, "What kind of self-respecting straight single man would go to a Belle and Sebastian concert?" Lots.

Your future boyfriend isn't there to make people think he's cool. He *is* cool, dammit. He's seen Beat Happening at the International Pop Underground three years in a row. He has the first pressing of their s/t album on vinyl. He is the college radio station DJ who is a legend to this day back at William and Mary. "Seriously, the photo of me and Morrissey is still on the wall in the station." He is the only one who "gets it." He is the proud owner of a vintage turntable that comes in its own suitcase. He is, of course, the biggest music snob you'll ever date and so in love with himself that you'll wonder if perhaps you're accidentally dating an artist again. Nah, he's not an artist but probably in publishing or some tragically low-paying but earnest profession. So, as with an artist, don't expect to be taken out to nice places.

If you think you're prepared for a life of being valued for your perceived taste in music, you must know what he holds dearest in the world. When he asks what other bands you're into, you say, "Oh, Felt, Architecture in Helsinki, Neutral Milk Hotel . . . too many to name, really! But my three favorite albums are *The Smiths*, *Tigermilk*, and *Pet Sounds*." Those three are the holy trinity. Learn them well. This will earn the instant approval of your new boyfriend and, even better, it might just get you a free drink. This is an achievement in and of itself with these boys.

And look! He's so sweet and sensitive. He'll tell you about his feelings. He'll communicate. There're songs he's (naturally) not afraid to cry to. In fact, he'll seek these out on the jukebox. This will cause embarrassment for you, but feel free to take this opportunity to go to the bathroom. He won't even notice you're gone. For the most part, he'll treat you well. Except when he scores tickets to Camera Obscura for your birthday instead of taking you to the restaurant with the two-month-long wait for reservations that you've been begging to go to, even if it means you'd have to pay.

Pros: Hey, finally someone you can share clothes with! And if he doesn't work out as a boyfriend, you've got a new gay BFF!

Cons: One day you will think you've progressed far enough in your relationship to admit that you like The Killers. You haven't. He will leave you. Wherever you are, he will leave you. If he has to stay an extra day in some random concert venue to avoid going back in the same car with the girl he thought he knew, he'll do it.

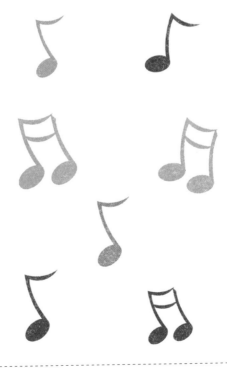

83

Go to Weddings

You can go through a lot of weddings in a short, hellish wedding season before you find a keeper. It's a tough game, this wedding business, but if you can keep yourself from getting too aggressive at the bouquet toss, throwing up on your shoes, or revealing your resentment toward yet another friend you'll never see again after her honeymoon, weddings are an ideal place to find your next boyfriend.

Chances are you're wearing a cringe-worthy bridesmaid dress, or are unnaturally squeezed into your prom dress. This might seem like a handicap, but in reality it works in your favor. There's nothing you can do about the petroleum-based fabric clinging unflatteringly about your person, and your future boyfriend knows this. He'll assume you look even better under normal circumstances, which may or may not be true.

The terrible cut/quality/color will be a kick start to your conversation. Once you start talking, though, you must be sure to be as gracious as possible. Whiny bridesmaid never won ride to the after party.

Much less a lasting relationship. Here are few lines that always work:

Him: That's quite the dress!

You: Yes, yes it is. [Smiling thinly] I'm always interested in trying out a new highly flammable material! Keep me away from those tea lights, won't you?

Him: [Laughs, offers arm] Let's go get drunk.

Or….

Him: Great job on that speech! I can't believe you kept a diary the entire time Kari and Tom were dating and that you brought the diary with you and that you wrote such thoughtful things about them.

You: [Surprised he fell for the oldest Maid of Honor trick in the book] Yes, they're so lucky to have me! I knew those two were made for each other since the first day they met. Which was . . . [Flip though fake diary] September 4, 2004. [Sigh]

Him: Let's go get a drink.

Or…

Him: Eek! That bouquet toss looked brutal!

You: Ha, yeah, I guess I've missed another one! If only I weren't so feminine and delicate and completely devoid of bloodlust. Say, would you mind terribly getting me something with ice in it for this black eye? It's beginning to swell.

Him: Oh, sure. Ice? Come on, let's go get a drink.

This, above all: don't let weddings get you down. No one wants to see you crying in the corner, reminiscing about how slutty the bride was in high school, or trying to put your hands in the groom's pocket. So take another sip of pinot grigio, plaster on that smile that you perfected during the rehearsal dinner, and be Emily Post in polyester.

Pros: Finally! You'll have a date for all those weddings you've got coming up!

Cons: You might change your mind about wanting to have a boyfriend in three months when your friends the new Dr. and Mrs. Brantley have become the two most boring people you've ever known.

84 Go to Oktoberfest

Munich is gorgeous that time of year, and you will be too, as far as the intoxicated Bavarians are concerned.

Call in sick to work for the week and hop the next Lufthansa flight to Deutschland. You won't regret it. Women, you see, like beer. But men like it a lot more. Lots. Oktoberfest is to them what the Barney's Warehouse Sale is to us. It's yet another one of those secret hiding places men go in droves. Follow them there and they will be delighted you did.

You'll have your pick of all ages, races, and nationalities. From locals who know the best tents to hit, to frat boys who fund-raised all year for this. Grab a stein, learn to rock blonde braids and a poofy skirt, and you've got it made, *meine Liebschen*.

Pros: You could meet Mr. Benz or Mr. BMW!

Cons: It's possible Freidrich is just *saying* that his last name is BMW. You'd better check his national identity card.

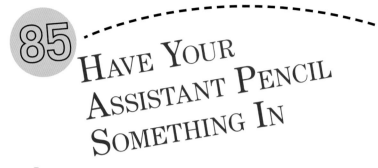

85 HAVE YOUR ASSISTANT PENCIL SOMETHING IN

Love your assistant? Hate her? **Either** way, it doesn't really matter, does it? She's got a job to do and that job is: make your life easier. Maybe "find boyfriend for boss" wasn't exactly in her job description. Maybe HR didn't mention that during her first interview. Maybe you didn't either. But there it is: you're a busy lady and nothing else seems to be working. It's time to start channeling Miranda Priestly. If your assistant's good, she'll come up with something. In these tough economic times (or if they're not, you'll see to it that they become so for her), it's hardly in her best interest to fail, now is it?

It works best to get on very well with your assistant. Find yourself a Girl Friday, always up for going the extra mile, rain or shine, whether or not she's fully recovered from the trichinosis she got when you accidentally threw away your clutch in the dumpster of that Chinese food place. To show her your appreciation, take her out for the occasional drink after work. She will repay generosity by bravely approaching men and explaining that her boss needs a lunch date—oh no, this wasn't her boss's idea at all! No, she's just really concerned about her boss because she's been doing nothing but work, work, work lately. Yes, that's her, over there, signing the check. Great hair, absolutely. So, could they pencil in something for next Tuesday? No, Wednesday? Great. She'll take his card so that she can confirm with his assistant on Monday. Lovely!

Isn't this a charming way to meet your new boyfriend? A little cowardly on your part, true, but best if he learns straightaway that you're a very busy and important person.

Pros: Your assistant knows all your favorite lunch places. At least you'll get your lobster ravioli.

Cons: Your assistant is adorable. Who's to say that men wouldn't be more interested in that plucky young thing than you?

86

GET A GIANT HDTV, PLAYSTATION 3, AND *ROCK BAND*

Send a text to all the single men in your phone saying you need help setting up your new equipment or choose a favorite guy for a more targeted approach. Paint your nails or mix yourself a drink while your new entertainment system (and your new electronics too) materializes before your eyes.

Pros: If for some reason it doesn't work out between you, who cares? You'll be too busy pretending to be a seventeen-year-old boy pretending to be Slash to notice your youth and good looks slowly draining away.

Cons: Your youth and good looks are slowly draining away.

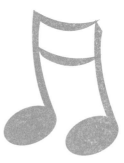

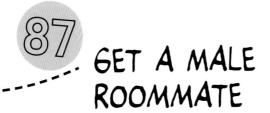

GET A MALE ROOMMATE

Living with a boy has its advantages. You'll have someone to get stuff down off the top shelves, he won't judge you for being a slob, he'll carry the heavy groceries, you'll have no passive-aggressive messages on the fridge, and you won't end up being on the same cycle! You'll also have access to all each other's friends and parties. He can provide you with an assortment of his coworkers and teammates for your consideration, and you can offer up your single girls. Soon it will be double dates around the clock. It's the best kind of mutual relationship.

Just resist the temptation to go for each other. This won't be hard once you've lived together for a while and you've seen how you live. You two are so disgusting! But no one else ever needs to know that.

Pros: And he'll kill all the spiders!

Cons: Resentment mounts after he's co-opted your friends and their parties and now no one needs you.

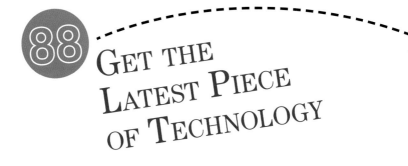

88

GET THE LATEST PIECE OF TECHNOLOGY

You're irresistible to all men* when you arrive on the scene with the newest piece of technology. They will immediately drop their books, cell phones, or last year's laptop to get an eyeful of what you're toting around. It's best if your employer can supply you with said latest piece of technology because then, when the men ask you about it as they start surrounding you like a herd of cats around a catnip mouse, you can say, "Yes, I suppose it is the new [repeat whatever he just said]. It's okay, I guess. I have no idea what it does." And then they will be off and running. Some will ask to hold it, some will ask how much it cost, and some will ask how old it is. It's like bringing an infant into a room full of college girls. Answer the questions to the best of your ability, or make it up as you go along.

*except Amish men

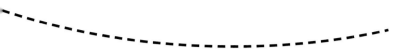

Pros: Every time you bring it out, you'll have a new set of phone numbers stored on it from men wanting to learn more about it. And you. Right, and you.

Cons: You have no idea how to access those numbers.

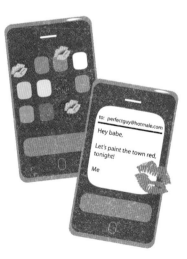

to: perfectguy@hotmale.com

Hey babe,

Let's paint the town red, tonight!

Me

89

TAKE GOLF LESSONS

Your mother was right: knowing how to golf is important. She was probably thinking more in terms of you finding a sport you could letter in and then one day having a better shot at climbing the corporate ladder, but that's okay, she doesn't have to know the real reason you've taken it up.

Taking golf lessons will tee you up for meeting a whole new class of future boyfriends. First there's the nice man in the pro shop who will sell you the latest set of Lady Cobras (the snake is scary, but they're pretty colors!) and help you coordinate your shoes with your glove and head covers. Then there's the pro assigned to teach you how to use the thousands of dollars of equipment you just bought. And after him come endless threesomes of men with whom you'll be hitting the links.

As you practice your newfound passion, all you have to do is be pleasant. And remember to keep your head down. And don't forget to downswing like you're ringing a bell. And for goodness' sake, keep your eyes in front of your hands. And make sure your right knee points toward the ball! There, that's all there is to it.

You shouldn't talk very much, so you're off the hook for thinking of anything that might interest your new golfing friends. (Though if you're caught behind a bachelor party or some other such annoying, slow-playing group, you will have to think of something to say. It should always pertain to golf. You can't go wrong if you stick to golf—talk about other courses, the new platinum-plated Titleists that have helium in the middle, or how Sergio Garcia is doing this year.) So turn on your cart and get ready to turn on all the single guys.

Pros: Golf fashion has come a long way. There are so many ways to look great out there!

Cons: Only one girl is going to give you any competition, but she's a formidable adversary: the drinks cart girl. Do not cross her.

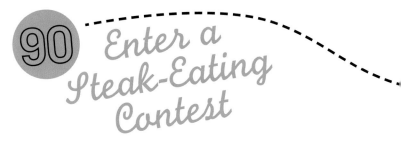

90 Enter a Steak-Eating Contest

Wow, a woman who's not afraid to eat! Who doesn't seem like she'd order a salad. Who would never beg you to take her to a vegan/raw/macrobiotic/all our meat was home-schooled organic restaurant. Who, in fact, is sitting in between two men three times the size of her with a seventy-two-ounce porterhouse in front of her. You (and the steak) will immediately

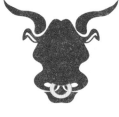

send them salivating, for behold: Woman. With Meat. You're appealing to their most primitive instincts. And aren't those your best bet anyway? Little point in appealing to the better angels of their nature, their sense of duty, or their higher selves.

Pros: You get to eat steak! As much as you possibly can eat, for one whole glorious meal of your life.

Cons: Ugh, you can't get fat! Boys hate women who love to eat but who also look like they've eaten. What a disgusting idea! Familiarize yourself with bulimia, the gym, or Adderall.

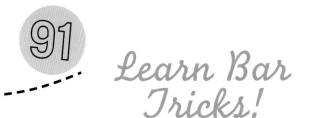

91. Learn Bar Tricks!

Coasters, salt shakers, maraschino cherries—they're all there for one thing: making you the life of the party. Use these common bar props to thrill and delight audiences of all ages and one gender. Are the natives getting restless? Stack a pint glass on top of another pint glass, rim to rim, with a coaster in between. Pull out the coaster quickly and wow one and all when the top pint glass is still balanced on the other! Pour salt onto the bar and balance a salt shaker on its edge. They won't see the little pile of salt keeping it balanced. Take the cherry from his Manhattan and tie the stem in a knot in your mouth.

It's not too different from babysitting except that your charges will buy you drinks and ask you out in return for your entertainment.

Pros: He'll be ordering you as many drinks that come with a garnish as he can think of.

Cons: Either that, or they'll burn you as a witch.

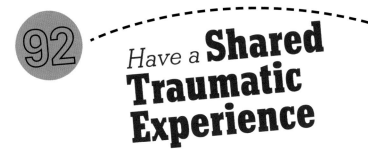

Have a **Shared Traumatic Experience**

Nothing brings people together like a traumatic experience! It will probably take some getting used to, but your first thought after something terrible or scary happens should always be, "Who's that guy over there who was in this with me and is he single?" Maybe you were both hostages at a bank heist, or maybe you were stuck in a cable car, high above the earth for twenty-four hours with nothing but half a bottle of water and an apple. Chat him up when you're both standing around with Red Cross blankets draped around you. Maybe his house and your house were the only two to be demolished in the most recent twister. Ask if he wants to get a cup of coffee down at the shelter! Perhaps you both transferred to the same university and have been treated like second-class citizens. Sit next to him in the back of the transfer bus! If it's looking like the end of the world because the polar ice cap melted and a tsunami has just hit New York and all of a sudden it's freezing and you're stuck in the New

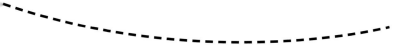

York Public Library burning their Gutenberg Bible for warmth, don't miss this great opportunity to put the moves on that dorky guy on your Academic Decathlon team with the hunky dad.

Traumatic experiences are all around you. Next time, instead of getting down about the unspeakable tragedy that just befell you, take it on the chin, catch him off guard, and get a date!

Pros: You'll always have your own little apocalypse.

Cons: You spent three weeks in a lifeboat with him. You don't think you've already exhausted everything interesting to talk about?

93

Go to Brooklyn, Even When You Don't Want To

There's a lot of merit in pulling it together. There are some nights you'd rather stay at home, or close to home, at least, and in comes an offer of a party in Brooklyn, or some other far-flung impossible-to-get-to part of the universe. It'd be so easy to say no. But guess what? You can't. When these things come up, you must say yes. You see, these are the times you will meet someone. It's not going to be when there's a little karaoke party right around the block from where you live that you'd planned to go to all week. Or when you've just gotten your hair blown out. It's when you're the most unmotivated to go that you're actually rewarded for your efforts. Just you watch.

Pros: It's so easy, once you get up, get dressed, and leave the house.

Cons: The guys you meet will live in Brooklyn or some other impossible location.

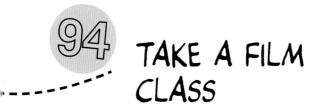

94 TAKE A FILM CLASS

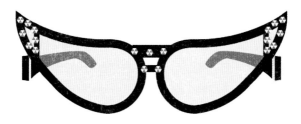

Don't know your Kurosawa from your Fellini? Think Eisenstein was a genius with silly hair and that montage was invented by the *Rocky IV* people? Take a film class to mitigate your shameful lack of cinema knowledge. You'll meet lots of guys in black who will be condescending at you until you've whipped yourself into shape. Or else they'll eat their shoe. You'd get that if you took a film class.

Pros: At least he'll stop talking at you once the movie's started.

Cons: You didn't like *Annie Hall*? You couldn't even finish it? *Oh my gosh, what is wrong with you? You don't know anything!*

95

Sponsor a Summer League Baseball Player

FAMILIES COME IN ALL SHAPES AND SIZES.

Some have a mom and a dad, some have only a mom, and some have two dads. Some kids are related to the rest of the family and some aren't. It doesn't make them any less of a family, because families are about love. If there's love, well, nothing else matters! Make this impassioned speech to the placement committee of your local summer league baseball team and you'll be leaving as a newly minted MILF for one very lucky college-age baseball player.

Summer league baseball is an institution in many parts of the U.S. The guys who play are promising young college kids who want to get more experience in while school is out. You can help them with that! The players are sometimes hometown heroes, but most are from out of state. Therefore, they need loving homes with generous families to stay with during the summer season. You can help them with that, too!

Most host families offer a traditional home away from home for these boys, complete with a host

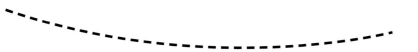

mom, host dad, host siblings, and host dog. Your guy might feel cheated at first, finding himself with only a host mom in a host one-bedroom apartment with a host pull-out couch, but soon he'll be the envy of his teammates and recognize how good he's got it. You'll be the super-cool mom sitting in the stands cheering him on and the super-hot hostess of all his post-game parties!

Pros: Lots of these kids go on to become professional baseball players. Surely when he's rich and famous, he won't forget the special (slightly older) lady who opened up her home to him and taught him how to run the bases in a completely different way.

Cons: The romance will end on the fifteenth day in a row of his requesting macaroni and cheese for dinner after you've finished washing another load of his jock straps.

96

DON'T WRITE A BOOK ABOUT HOW TO FIND A BOYFRIEND

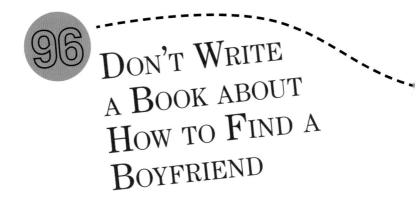

You'll have a lot more Saturday nights free if you're not stuck inside with your laptop and the rest of your roommate's bottle of red wine, working your fingers to the bone, racing against a deadline.

Pros: You'll be living it, not writing about it.

Cons: You might not have thought of it if you weren't getting paid for it.

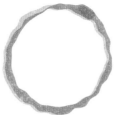

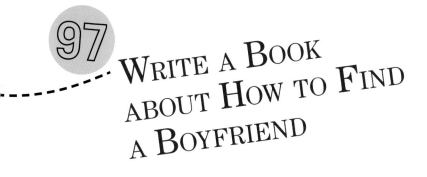

97 WRITE A BOOK ABOUT HOW TO FIND A BOYFRIEND

Most people, even men who don't read, think books are serious and important.

Tell him you are writing a book and he'll be happy to help with the research, even if it's about something very trivial. Even better if it's about something very trivial. Maybe there will be something in it for him. Maybe you'll use his name, or the name of his cat who died too soon. Perhaps he'll get a shout out in the acknowledgments. He'll stick around at least until your publication date to find out.

Pros: That's one more sale of your book! Ka-ching!

Cons: The book launch party will be a "This Is Your Life" of all the questionable decisions you've ever made.

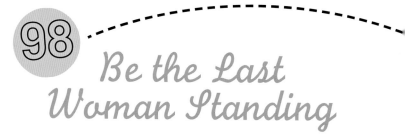

98

Be the Last Woman Standing

The brilliance of this one is that it works both in the literal and the abstract. Take a night out. It's getting later and later and everyone's getting sloppier and sloppier, except you. There could be any number of reasons for this, from performance-enhancing drugs, to your preternaturally high tolerance for hard alcohol, or maybe you've finally smartened up and started alternating pints of water with shots of bourbon. (Ha ha, right.)

At any rate, they're falling down around you, particularly the ladies and the Asian men. And you've kept your cool. Well done, you! This will score well with the frat boys, country boys, and European intelligentsia.

It's three in the morning, but you're still in fine form to go back to his place to play beer pong, or go to the truck stop for a grilled cheese and hash browns, or head to that little wine bar to talk Camus and smoke Gauloises. So what if there were smarter, thinner, and prettier girls back there, four hours ago? They're gone now!

And here you are and there he is, and once he gets to see how great you are, away from the teeming masses, that's the end of the story. All because you outlasted the rest of them.

And, as for the rest of your life . . .

Let's not kid ourselves: this whole time it had nothing to do with you. Men will settle down when they feel like it, and all the goddesses in the world can cross their paths, but if it's before their genetically preordained time, they won't look twice at you. But, if you're at the right place at the right time, you're golden.

Maybe all your friends and relatives have had the good (or bad, you saw how it ended for Cousin Rhea) fortune to have found someone to spend the next five to ten years with and you're still on the shelf. Big deal. Just be patient and wait it out.

You won't be single forever or else you won't be unhappily single forever. Either way you win. And isn't that what it's all about?

Pros: To love one's self is to begin a lifelong romance, wrote Oscar Wilde. Cultivate that relationship and you'll never be lonely again.

Cons: You'll need to find something to do while you're waiting for the end of the night or for the male population of the world to come around. You may as well go out there and try to find a boyfriend. Just for fun, mind you, for the sake of adventure and living it up before you're saddled with dependent humans and your carefree days are gone. Go be fabulous.

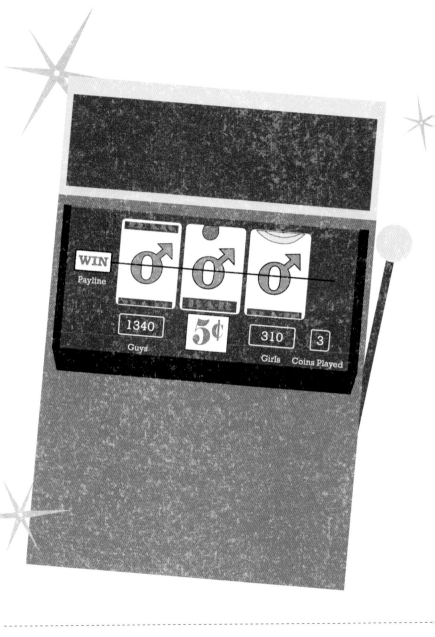

ACKNOWLEDGMENTS

So many talented people were enormously helpful during the creation of this book. My editor, Ann Treistman, provided direction and creativity, without which I would have been lost. Designer LeAnna Weller Smith and illustrator Tamela Parton created a gorgeous package that will continue to delight me years after this has published. The super sharp Rosemary Counter and Jen Brazas lent their extraordinary talents early on. And of course I wouldn't be anywhere without Sam Hiyate, agent extraordinaire.

Family and friends, I love you. Aaron Berth forgot he played a key role. Megan Buckley and Peter Guy cheered from across the ocean. Martha Josephson repeated everything I said back to me. Signe Pike communed with the fairies. Abby Plesser commiserated. Lea Beresford was an energizing ray of sunshine. Lizzie Batey Yoder was a font of stellar ideas (it's no wonder she's landed a doctor). Karissa Ellis Singleton provided turkey soup. My colleagues at work, who are used to having their names in print, were heartwarmingly supportive. Chryse Heckman kept me in fiestatinis. Both Morris Tang and my roommate provided male perspectives. Stephanie Higgs was my fairy godsister.

My family pulled it together beautifully: My father supplied a fantastic number of suggestions and a heap of encouragement. My sister Jennifer gave me all her best politically incorrect material (not appearing in this book). My mother kept me from going off the deep end and pretty much made everything possible from day one.